Chapter One – April 2016

4.18.2016

OK...Let's make it official. My beautiful bride, Judy, has been diagnosed with Acute Lymphoblastic Leukemia today. We're waiting on an additional test this afternoon to determine if the Philadelphia chromosome is positive or negative. This will determine the course of action and treatment plan. Once determined, the treatment will start immediately.

Last week, she was exhibiting systems of flu. General body aches, low grade temperature, no appetite. We got her in to our Internist Dr. Lawrence Lee on Wednesday. Flu swab was negative and he did a lab blood panel workup and called back on Thursday with preliminary results. Thursday and Friday, Judy just felt progressively worse. On Friday afternoon, Dr. Lee, in consultation with the Hematology/Oncology department at Brookwood, determined that we should bring her to UAB due to the extremely high White Blood Cell count, low platelet count and the opportunity to have additional diagnostic tests run that weren't available at Brookwood. We were admitted through the ER Friday afternoon and the care has been nonstop since.

6
Unidades.

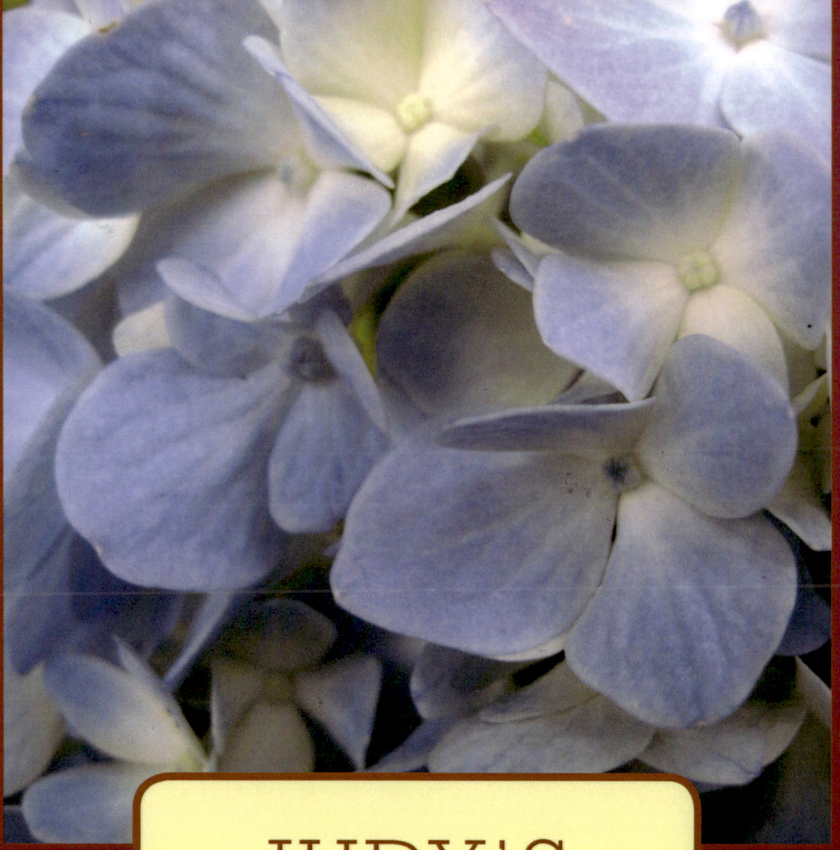

JUDY'S JOURNEY

A WALK OF FAITH THROUGH A BATTLE WITH LEUKEMIA

RICK McCOY

Forward

From August 2015 through December 2016, our senior pastor at Hunter Street Baptist Church, Buddy Gray, led our congregation in an emphasis on living *coram Deo*, a Latin phrase literally meaning "before God." For centuries, theologians have used this phrase to describe life in the presence of God, understanding that we live every moment of our lives under God's watchful gaze and sovereign care. Living *coram Deo* means living one's entire life in the presence of God, under the authority of God, to the glory of God.

On April 13, 2016, Judy McCoy, a longtime active member of Hunter Street, went to see her internist with symptoms of the flu - aches, a low-grade fever, and a loss of appetite. Two days later she was admitted to the hospital, diagnosed with Acute Lymphocytic Leukemia. That began a whirlwind year of chemo treatments, infusions, venipunctures, lumbar punctures, bone marrow biopsies, radiation treatments, the hope of remission, bone marrow transplant, chest tubes, feeding tubes, O2 Oxygen, the devastation of recurrence, clinical trials, travel to Houston, and ultimately on Good Friday, 2017, Judy's transition from death to eternal life in the presence of her Lord with her family by her side.

Prior to her diagnosis, Judy had lived *coram Deo*, encouraging and ministering to her co-workers, serving the church joyfully and faithfully, and mentoring countless young women. After her diagnosis, Judy continued to live *coram Deo*, facing each experience of suffering with an authentic, radiant faith in Jesus Christ that drew others to her. One of her oncology nurses made these remarks that I read at her memorial service: "Judy personified the inexplicable, supernatural joy that can only be found in Jesus. This joy and hope she found in Him was evident to anyone who had a conversation with her, even in her darkest times. Her joy was evident in her demeanor with her bright smile, facial expressions, and kind mannerisms. It was evident in her outlook as she bravely faced a devastating disease with a hope and joy that rose above the disease and calamity within her physical body. It was evident in her interactions. She listened intently and made each person feel special and important. Judy made a point to address everyone by name and ask how their day was with genuine concern. She shared her joy with doctors and environmental service employees alike. She was the kind of person who made everybody feel like somebody. I can confidently say Judy is now experiencing the ultimate joy as she is in the presence of Jesus, her Lord and Savior, healed and whole."

Christians do not seek out suffering, but we understand it is a universal experience of all living in this fallen world. And more than that, we trust the Scriptural evidence that God works redemptively in our suffering, deepening our relationship with Him (Job 42:5, Psalm 73:25-26), developing our spiritual maturity (Romans 5:3-5, James 1:2-4), equipping us to minister to others (2 Corinthians 1:3-4), and providing an opportunity to glorify God through our persevering faith (1 Peter 1:6-9, Revelation 7:13-17). Judy's resilient joy was not based in her circumstances but in her relationship with her Savior.

She endured her path of suffering with the confident hope Paul expressed in Romans 8:17b-18: "[W]e suffer with [Christ] in order that we may also be glorified with him. For I consider that the sufferings of this present time are not worth comparing with the glory that is to be revealed to us." Judy shone the light of Christ into every space she moved and inspired all who knew her, in life and in death.

Throughout Judy's journey, her husband Rick was by her side. Thirty-five years before Judy's diagnosis, Rick stood at a church altar and promised to love his wife in sickness and in health. His steadfast commitment to his vows as he walked arm-in-arm with Judy through the dark valley of the Shadow of Death should serve as an example for all husbands of how to treat your wife with honor and love her sacrificially. When the bone marrow transplant required an extended hospitalization spanning many months, Rick stayed with Judy the entire time. He manufactured a bed out of the uncomfortable chair in the small room and some extra padding, spent many hours grilling physicians and researching all options for her treatment, and consistently comforted and encouraged the love of his life as she endured the horrors of her disease and accompanying treatment. It was a gracious gift of God to allow me to witness the love, courage, and faith of this remarkable couple on display in an extraordinarily difficult season.

Soon after Judy's diagnosis, Rick began chronicling her journey on the Caring Bridge website. Rick's posts on Caring Bridge became appointment reading, not only for his updates on Judy, but for the wit, humor, honesty, and poignancy that marked his words, always pointing to our hope in Christ and ending with the reminder to live *coram Deo*. I am thrilled he has undertaken the hard but important task of reflecting on Judy's journey and writing this book.

As you read the pages herein, I pray you will be challenged and inspired by Judy's journey as I have been. May you see the glory of Christ and be emboldened to walk by faith through whatever circumstances you must endure. And may you hold fast to the truth expressed in 1 Peter 1:6-7: "In this you rejoice, though now for a little while, if necessary, you have been grieved by various trials, so that the tested genuineness of your faith – more precious than gold that perishes though it is tested by fire – may be found to result in praise and glory and honor at the revelation of Jesus Christ. "

CORAM DEO

Brian Hinton
Associate Pastor
Hunter Street Baptist Church

Judy's Journey

Judy McCoy was the wife of Rick McCoy and mother to Matt and Jennifer. In April of 2016, she was diagnosed with ALL, Acute Lymphoblastic Leukemia. It is rare to see this form of pediatric leukemia in adults. After 2 rounds of failed chemotherapy and 2 successful rounds of a targeted antibody therapy at the University of Alabama at Birmingham, Judy was presented for a Bone Marrow Transplant in October of 2016.

Unfortunately, a bone marrow biopsy performed in early February 2017 showed that her leukemia had relapsed. Judy traveled to MD Anderson in Houston, TX for a referral appointment in late February 2017 to possibly participate in a clinical trial.

Throughout the process, Judy remained firm in her faith and continues to be an inspiration to all she met. She said that if going through all this leads even just one person to the Lord, it will have all been worth it.

This is her story…

Judy's Journey

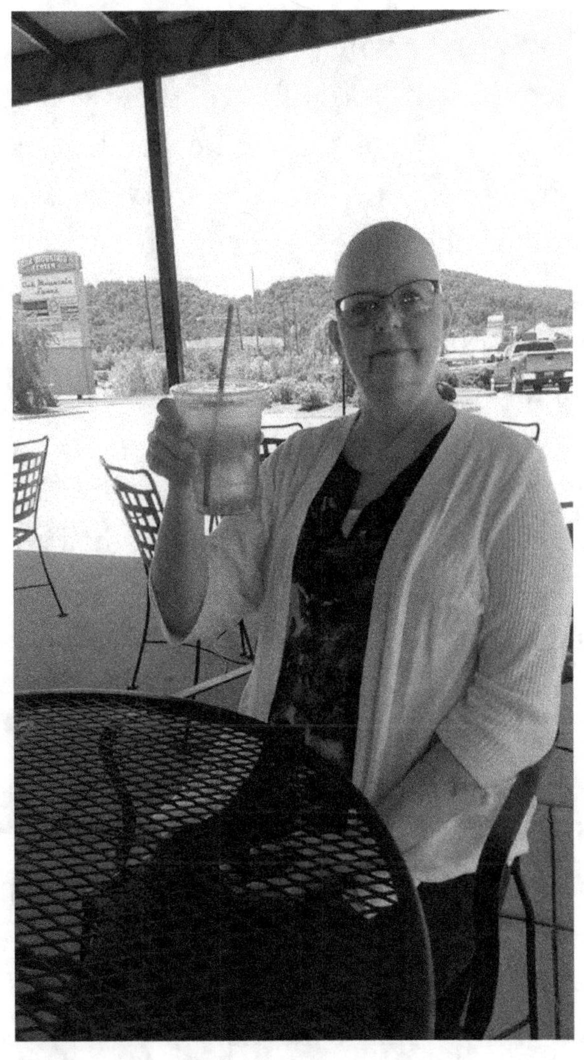

A walk of faith through a battle with leukemia

Rick McCoy

Pain management is under control by alternating a couple of different types of meds. Still no appetite to speak of. She is resting comfortably and sleeping quite a bit. (The meds are really really really good!!!)

We are currently on the Bone Marrow Transplantation unit due to the monitoring available and the critical nature she was in upon arrival. Since the regiment of meds has the WBC headed in the correct direction and having received a couple of units of platelets (one yesterday and one today), we will be moved to the Hematology/Oncology floor as early as this afternoon or tomorrow morning to begin treatment.

We covet your prayers as we begin this journey. We know the Great Physician and know He has Judy's name written in the palm of His hand. We are so thankful for the staff's knowledge, training and compassionate care. Please pray specifically for Dr. Mehta and his Nurse Practitioner Laura Romundstad.

Stay tuned for more! Coram DEO

4.19.2016 Update

Still waiting on the gene test to determine the treatment plan. Doctor is expecting it this afternoon. Nurse Practitioner thinks it may be tomorrow. Please pray for sooner rather than later. Judy is sleeping a lot due to the pain meds, but pain is running between 2 and 7 depending on timing. Coram DEO

4.20.2016 Update

Still waiting. One of the Docs called the lab this morning while they were on rounds and lab indicated we would have results this afternoon. So...still waiting! Coram DEO

4.20.2016 17:00 Update

YES...YES...YES...Praise God from Whom all blessings flow! The gene test came back negative which means that Judy can start chemo very soon. We will be meeting with a clinical trial director tomorrow to see if Judy qualifies to be a participant. Either way, we now have a path to follow.

We are so confidant in the UAB staff, from the lead doctors, to nurses, to Mike who cleans our room. They are absolutely the best, sweetest spirited people we've ever had the pleasure to meet. (Just wish it was a tiny bit better circumstances!)

We are confident in this, that He Who began a good work in us will bring it to completion. Coram DEO

4.21.2016 Update

Lots and lots of progress. We met with Dr. Harry Erba this morning around 08:00 to discuss the possibility of Judy participating in a clinical trial. He felt like she was a good candidate. We have reviewed the research trial paperwork and have signed the consent forms. Additional blood tests and bone marrow tests are being conducted as I type this. We'll know by tomorrow if she is approved for the trial. Either way, Judy will start chemo tomorrow. Coram DEO

4.22.2016 Update

The clinical trial is not a blind trial. During the initial induction phase of the chemo, a computer will randomly pick if a participant will receive the test drug or not. Either way, the same regiment of drugs will continue. We will know if she is picked as the additional drug will be introduced. This drug is already FDA approved. It is not given unless a patient has initially entered remission and has had a relapse. Because this drug has such a good success rate during a second induction, the focus of the trial is to see if introduction of the drug during the initial induction produces better remission results for the long term.

Pray for God's direction for inclusion or not in the clinical trial. Pray for Dr. Harry Erba, Director of Hematology Malignancy Program & Professor of Hematology/Oncology at UAB School of Medicine. Also Angel Elliott, Research Nurse Coordinator. We want the results to bring glory to Him and Him alone. If this valley that we're currently in will prevent someone else from walking this path, then, bring it. We can handle all things through Christ who gives us strength. Coram DEO

4.22.2016 15:00 Update

You know how it feels to be loved and accepted? John 3:16 is an excellent example of the greatest love that could ever be known. Another is the love that Judy & I have felt since this journey began coming from you, our friends and family. We are blown away by the offers to come sit with Judy, cut our grass, run errands, cards, texts and yes...in Judy's case...a box of chocolates. Do you know how it feels to be accepted? We do because...

JUDY'S BEEN ACCEPTED TO THE CLINICAL TRIAL!!!!!!!!

We are so thankful that this trial will produce results that can possibly help future leukemia patients. The chemo induction phase will start this afternoon. Please pray for Judy's tolerance of the drugs, stamina for the induction phase and a positive reaction to the treatment. Coram DEO

4.22.2016 21:00 Update

OK. For all you techie types...get ready. This is for our prayer warriors that like to use specific info in their prayers. For those of you (like me this past week) that can only groan through your prayers right now, the following will probably make your eyes roll back into your head!

Judy is participating in "A Phase III Randomized Trial of Blinatumomab for Newly Diagnosed BCR-ABL negative B lineage Acute Lymphoblastic Leukemia in Adults". Judy was asked to take part because she is between the ages of 30 & 70 and recently diagnosed with a subtype of acute lymphoblastic leukemia (ALL) that is known as BCR-ABL negative B-lineage ALL. The drug therapies utilized throughout the trial are (not all at the same time): Cytarabine, Daunorubicin, Vincristine, Dexamethasone, Methotrexate, Pegaspargase, Cyclophosphamide, Cytarabine, 6 Mercaptopurine, Leucovorin, Blinatumomab, Etoposide, Prednisone, and a partridge in a pear tree.

Infusion will begin around 9 tonight. Stay tuned for more! Coram DEO

4.23.2016 Update

When you hear people talk about the 'C' word. What's your first thought? Yeah...this week 'cancer' has come to the forefront of our thoughts as well. But what we want to focus on and are striving to focus on is the 'C' word that provides the greatest healing available. That word is evidenced in the name of 'Christ'. He and He alone is our Sustenance and Sustainer. He brought Judy through her first two infusions of chemo last night pain free. No nausea. No aches. Woke up at 4:00 this morning and was actually hungry. Ate a better breakfast than she's eaten in a week. Has showered. Fresh pajamas. Put war paint on and is ready for the day. We're about to go cruising the hallways because she feels like it. That's either the hard-headed Langston blood or the professional Physical Therapist coming out. (Not sure which but I have my suspicions). Judy sure has a new respect for the acute patients that she's dealt with for years. She has an empathy now that has replaced sympathy for her patients. She truly knows how they feel.

Doctor Mehta came in on rounds this morning and was extremely pleased in her progress over the last two days. He told her to rejoice in the daily victories and that's exactly what we've doing. To Him that is able...we praise You and thank You for these victories. Coram DEO

4.24.2016 Update

Third Day. It's our favorite Southern Rock Band. We've followed them for years. Love their lyrics, passion and live shows. The lead singer, Mac Powell, has a very distinctive voice that just cradles you like a warm Mother's hug. (pretty sappy huh?)

Third Day. It's also the number of days that Judy has felt incredibly well for what she's going through. The routine is sleep, pee, sleep, pee, repeat. I'm really interested to know how many bags of IV saline she's gone through so far. Her appetite is coming back a little more each day. This morning she ate all her eggs, sausage patty, fresh fruit cup, and about 10 bites of granola with yogurt mixed in. All washed down with coffee. Those of you that know Judy know that when she started wanting coffee again...well, that's a very good sign. So thankful for this strength building time as we know there will be some very tough days ahead during this journey.

Third Day. It's how long our Lord & Savior, Jesus Christ, laid in the tomb before rising. Just as He said He would. He did that so that we dirty, filthy, rotten, fully loved people could have an advocate that knows our fears, hopes, aspirations, concerns, and uncertainties. He did that so that if we put our faith and hope in Him, then someday our faith will become sight and we will behold Him in all of His glory. We sincerely hope & pray you know this peace that passes all understanding.

We appreciate so much the out pouring of love, prayers and concern for Judy and me. The cards, texts, FB messages, prayers, visits, and calls truly uplift her and carry her forward. We feel so loved and please know that it is truly felt. Coram DEO

4.24.2016 20:30 Update

Another really good day today. Very low pain. Showered. Personal clothes instead of the stylish hospital gowns with the peak-a-boo back side opening. Excellent appetite. We've walked the halls. Watched Shrek 2 on the in-room DVD player. Took an afternoon nap because our pastor says all the Godly people take Sunday afternoon naps.

Please keep Judy in your continued prayers for tomorrow morning. She will be having a lumbar puncture early in the morning. This will produce a baseline for the spinal fluid as well as test the fluid for any leukemia cells. They will also be injecting one of the chemo drugs directly into the spinal fluid. She'll have to remain still for 2 hours post procedure and possible side effects are severe headache and nausea. We'd like for those side effects to be non-existent.

Thanks again for lifting her to our Father. He still hears and answers. Coram DEO

4.25.2016 Update

This morning, Judy had the lumbar puncture and came through it with flying colors. No pain. No nausea. No spinal headache. She is defying the odds and we sure know why. The Great Physician is guiding and directing the entire medical staff. We praise Him for their knowledge, wisdom, compassion, understanding, words of encouragement, etc, etc, etc. Nurses that Judy has had on the floor that have been off and then rotated back on to other patients are all stopping me in the hallway to inquire how she's doing. She continues to touch people's hearts in the midst of walking her journey. Faith for the Journey. She shines it every day. Coram DEO

4.26.2016 Update

How do you start to say thank you for the overwhelming support, love, cards, phone calls, visits, goodie bags, pizza parties, errand offers, grass trimming, weed whacking, clothes washing, spend the night parties, scripture books, magazines, and most of all...DARK CHOCOLATE that we have received from you, our family and dear friends. All we can think to say is that y'all are truly the hands and feet of Christ. You have blown us away with the way that you rally around us. I'm sure that if you listen for the still, small voice that you'll hear "Well done, good and faithful servant".

Judy continues to string very good days together. She has still not experienced any nausea or headaches from any of the chemo treatments. This is truly an answer to the prayers that you are offering on her behalf. We continue to feel and appreciate the prayers of His children.

Please pray that Judy will continue to gain strength each day. The first week here really depleted her energy due to the severe pain that she was dealing with. (9 and 10 on a constant 24 hour a day basis). She has not had any pain medication since last Friday afternoon! Please also pray that all of the paperwork will be completed in a timely manner to apply for short and long term disability as well as her medical insurance claims. Pray that my work schedule will coordinate with my need to be at the hospital to support Judy when she needs me to be here. We love and appreciate y'all. Coram DEO

4.27.2016 Update

Judy has come to the realization that she can't eat dark chocolate pretzels and then have her blood sugar taken about 30 minutes later. Yesterday and today her blood sugar spiked. Nothing that has the medical staff concerned because she has been receiving steroid medicine as part of her treatment and this will elevate her levels anyway. The medicine, combined with her love of dark chocolate, just elevated it a bit more. So...the chocolate has been relegated to the closet until the steroids are stopped which we think tomorrow is the final treatment for this phase. Just wanted everyone to know in case you come to visit and she's in a 'roid rage' and wants to hit you with a WWE Raw folding chair.

She's been really fatigued today but still PAIN FREE!!!!!!! Appetite has been fair, but she's still trying to fill the pie hole on her good days. She's really enjoying visitors and loves seeing everyone. We ask that no flowers or live plants be sent as her immune system is fragile at the moment and these can be triggers for reaction. She truly loves the cards and baked goodies. Every single day a staff member from our church has visited and/or called. We are so very blessed with a loving, caring church family. We love y'all. Coram DEO

4.28.2016 Update

Three Little Words - I love you.

Simple words that really kick-start a relationship. Words to build a lifetime together upon. Words that lead you down an aisle-way to voice a set of vows that proclaim that you'll never leave or forsake each other. Through sickness and health, richer or poorer. Life's ups and downs. Mountain tops and the deepest valleys. Judy's been on the mountaintop today. Great pain free day where she showered and dressed herself. Sat in the room chair for ~ 4 hours. Cruised the hallways for a lap around the nurse's station. Excellent appetite. Visited with family. Really a perfect day except for being confined to the hospital.

Three Little Words - You have leukemia.

More complex words that really have a way of turning your world upside down. Words that create hundreds of questions that seemingly have no answers. How? Why? Did we miss indicators? What's the treatment look like? Will I lose my hair? Will I live? Who will stand with us? Who may run? How are we going to handle all of our obligations? And based on all these questions...the answers may or may not come. But that's where our faith comes in to play. Faith that we professed to each other in front of family and friends years ago. Faith to stand with each other no matter what life throws at us. Faith in our God that He loves us, cares for us, and will send the correct answer at exactly the correct time.

Three Little Words - It is finished.
The final words that Christ said as He gave up His last breath. Final words that bridge the gap once and for all for those that believe. Words that give hope of a brighter tomorrow. Words that show how very much He loves us and desires a relationship with us. Words that teach us how to treat each other and to look out for each other when life throws its curve balls at us. Words that our friends and family are living out each and every day. We truly love you for loving us. Coram DEO

4.30.2016 Update

Well...leukemia reared its ugly head yesterday. As mentioned on Wednesday, Judy had her last steroid treatment on Thursday and had not taken any pain medication since last Friday the 22nd. Dr. Mehta had mentioned earlier this week that the steroids were really helping with her pain management. So...throughout yesterday Judy's back pain started coming back. She thought it was just back spasms at first but as the night progressed, the pain continued to escalate. When her night nurse came in to start her Friday night chemo treatment, she was really in a lot of pain. She finally took a morphine injection to control the pain enough to receive the chemo and then an oxycodone tablet to rest the remainder of the night. This morning she is achy but not in the severe pain of last night.

The chemo treatment has been tolerated just like last week's treatment. No nausea and no headache. We are very thankful for this. Please continue to pray for us as we try to learn how to deal with the daily ups and downs of this disease. Rejoice with us in the daily victories that come from answered prayers. We truly appreciate your prayers, cards, texts and calls. Y'all are simply the best. Coram DEO

Chapter Two – May 2016

5.1.2016 Update

This is the day that the Lord has made. We will rejoice and be glad in it!

We're learning the ups and downs of living with Judy's leukemia. She's learning to stay ahead of the pain curve and use all of the tools available in her tool kit to combat and win over this disease. Her care continues to be absolutely top shelf. We are so blessed in this town to have a world class facility right here. When we've researched her care team, we've come to realize that they are some of the most talented clinicians in their field with pedigrees from the world's finest institutions. Yale, Harvard, Stanford Medical School, All India Institute of Medical Sciences, City of Hope Hospital, Medical College Baroda, LSU Medical School, Johns Hopkins, UAB Medical School, and the list goes on and on. These pedigrees combined with your prayers on our behalf are truly lifting Judy towards a full and complete remission.

And He and He alone will receive the glory, honor and praise. Coram DEO

5.2.2016 Update

What a great day! Judy said this is the best day she's had since being admitted. Sat in the chair after breakfast and shower until around mid-afternoon. We both learned a valuable lesson on Friday about staying ahead of the pain. She's managed much better since then. We continue to be blown away with the love and support that y'all are sending our way. Thank you. Thank you.

Prayer requests for this week are (1) that Judy's digestive system will work a little better. Some of the medicines she takes lead to a bit of constipation and the solutions for that need to work a little quicker and better. (2) She will have another lumbar puncture on Friday morning that will place chemo into her spinal column/fluid. Pray that she will react as positively as she did to the first one. No headache and no nausea. (3) Her Friday night chemo treatment of both medicines to be tolerated as well as the first two. Again...no nausea.

Judy continues to touch the UAB staff as she walks this journey. Nurses that have rotated off continue to pop in to check on her and just to visit. Her faith is amazing to see in action. To God be the glory, great things He has done. Coram DEO

5.4.2016 Update

Happy Star Wars Day everyone! Judy celebrated by making **2** laps around the hallway this afternoon. Moved faster than she has in days. Got up this morning and unplugged her IV from the wall socket, went across the hallway to the coffee pot, and fixed her own coffee! Each day brings new mercies for which we are grateful. We expect pretty uneventful days until Fridays. Friday is usually when she will get her chemo treatments and they are around the 9:00 hour. This Friday, she will get a lumbar puncture early Friday morning and her chemo treatment that night, so, she could really use your prayers for no headache, no nausea and no pain. Thank y'all so very much for lifting her to our Father. He is listening and answering. Coram DEO

5.5.2016 Update

Where do I even begin? How about with a prayer of praise and thanksgiving? Judy found out this morning that if her blood levels continue on the current path and if they stabilize over the next week, it's entirely possible that she'll get to come home for a week on Day 22 of this saga! That would be Friday the 13th. What a day of rejoicing that will be! She'll be able to come home to her own house, her own bed, her own dogs, and even her own husband. What a great week that will be. She'll still need to return for continued treatment, but WOW, what a rapid change of events.

Thank you Lord for your continued healing of our precious Judy. Thank You that You are always faithful towards us and hold us in the palm of your hand. Thank You for being the Great Physician. Coram DEO

5.7.2016 Update

Judy's lumbar puncture (LP) yesterday morning went well. She had her first bout of very mild nausea that passed quickly. I feel like it was brought on by the chemo meds injected during the LP and moving her from the procedure room back to her room here on the 7th floor. The LP meds were some of the strongest yet, but once about an hour had passed, she was great for the remainder of the day. No spinal headache from the LP procedure! She had absolutely no side effects from the chemo treatment last night. So overall, she is an absolute trooper for having 2 separate treatments in the same day. Judy's really looking forward to seeing her kids tomorrow on Mother's Day. They've been so good about visiting and checking on her every day. Jennifer has been dealing with a case of the sniffles this past week so she has stayed away from the hospital but has checked on her Momma daily. Matt comes up and lets us watch him eat supper. It's the highlight of our day. (Not really).

We say this a lot but we truly are blessed by you, our family & friends, for the way that you are upholding us with your prayers, cards, telephone calls, visits, meals, fresh baked goodies, gift cards, and the list goes on and on. Thank you for loving us through this journey. Coram DEO

5.8.2016 Update

Mother's Day in the hospital. Not what we were expecting a few weeks ago. Judy, like most moms, just wants to see her kids on Mother's Day. It can be over a home cooked meal, a restaurant, worshiping together in church, or just hanging out like we got to do today. Matt, Charlie, Jennifer, & Phillip came up to the hospital and surprised their Momma with a Dairy Queen Chocolate Extreme Blizzard, some new lounging pajamas, and a couple of coloring books and gel pens. But spending time together with our adult children is what's good for her soul right now.

Judy is a little fatigued today, but was feeling that way before the family visits. The doctor came in on rounds this morning and stated that they are very pleased with how far she has come in such a short time. She continues to respond favorably to the chemo treatments. She is starting to notice a few more stray hairs on her shirts and brushes so she is ready for the loss of her hair. She's discussed it with our niece that has been doing her hair and they've decided to cut it all off when she's ready and go with pretty scarves and/or do rags. She received a couple of really beautiful scarves from Jen & Phillip's trip to Disney with the Helena Band.

We were able to watch our church's live stream this morning and really appreciate the technology that makes that possible. Seeing our friends and neighbors worshiping made us feel right at home. Just wish we could have been there instead of here. But here is where we are. We are looking so forward to the opportunity to maybe go home next Saturday for a week break from treatments. I know the dogs will be as excited to see Judy as she is to see them.

Your prayers continue to be heard and answered. You bless us each time you lift us to the throne room of our gracious loving God. Thank you. Coram DEO

5.9.2016 Update

What does Coram DEO mean? I've tried to close each of our updates with this Latin phrase. My junior high Latin teacher, Ms. McCollum, would be so proud. Especially since 'ego amo te' is about all I recall from her class. But back to the original question that we've gotten since this journey began. What does it mean?

Coram DEO translated means before the face of God. The idea of the Christian life means to live one's entire life in the presence of God, under the authority of God, to the glory of God. This has been the underlying theme of our study at our church this year. It means to realize that everything we do should have an overarching realization that our very existence, lives, work, family, relationships, worship, recreation, prayers, needs, wants, desires should be lived out with the thought that God is wanting an intimate relationship with us, His ultimate creation. To live in the presence of God should be at the forefront of our thoughts to ultimately bring glory to Him and Him alone.

Do Judy and I live this out every day? She comes much closer than I do, but it is the goal of our lives to strive towards living Coram DEO. To treat others the way we want to be treated. To love God and love others. To reflect the very presence of the Living God in our lives, to surrender our lives to His direction, and to give Him the honor and glory due His Name.

The doctor rounds this morning confirmed that she is doing exceptionally well in response to her treatments. If blood work continues to improve then plans are underway to let Judy come home this weekend for at least a week, possibly two. That just blows our minds that she has responded this well and this quickly. To God be the glory, great things He has done. Coram DEO

5.10.2016 Update

Today's edition of Judy's Journey finds us learning to understand nausea. It seems to rear its ugly head without any prior warning (most of the time). We were in the middle of a conversation yesterday and a wave of nausea hit her mid-sentence. Thankfully the trusty bucket was nearby. The wave lasts about a minute and then it's gone. Laura, her CRNP, said this morning she was surprised that Judy had not experienced more nausea than she had to date. Judy is learning to utilize Zofran throughout the day as needed to help control the nausea. So...please pray that the nausea will subside and the chemo continue to be well tolerated.

The lab work continues to show improvement and talks are still underway to get her home this weekend for a break in the treatment schedule. Pray also for her fatigue level. She gets fatigued very easily but each day the recovery time is getting quicker.

The cards, visits, calls and texts are such great medicine for the soul. We appreciate each and every one of them and are truly blessed that you are loving on us daily. We love y'all. Coram DEO

5.12.2016 Update

I don't like it when I don't get to see her. Today at work, one of my co-workers had nausea and vomiting. (I asked her if this was sympathy symptoms for Judy). And so…in the interest of not wanting to even suspect that I've caught and/or are carrying the nausea germ, I will stay away from Judy for 24 hours just to make sure. Her immune system is so severely compromised due to her leukemia that she has nothing with which to fight even the smallest of infections. So I'll err on the side of caution.

Judy received a different type of nausea medication last night (Fioracett) and it has done the trick for her so far. She's received another unit of blood today and has done really well. The decision will be made probably late tomorrow if she will be able to come home for a week for a break in the treatment plan. But the main thing is to make sure that she is strong enough and safe enough to come home for even a little break. We'll rely on the doctor's good judgment (and God's direction) for that time frame.

Judy has a wonderful friend that had our house cleaned today by a professional maid service. What an awesome gift to have a clean house for her to come home to when the time is right. I've been duly threatened by this friend that the house better still be clean when Judy comes home. I'm thinking of sleeping in the truck till then. This friend is just another example of the way God has used His people to support us in and through this journey. We are truly blessed that you love us as He loves us. Coram DEO

5.14.2016 Update

Judy's chemo treatment last night was well tolerated. No headache or nausea this morning. Plans are still underway to get her released home and the new target date is now Monday the 16th. But we want to make sure that she's medically stable enough to go home. A couple of more days to ensure that her headaches and nausea are under control are what we are praying for. Fatigue is still an issue, but as her blood responds to the treatments and continues to level out, this will get better as well.

Let me say something about the community we live in. We moved to Pelham 24 years ago. Our children were raised there. I've been fortunate to have worked a good amount of that time for companies that are headquartered or based in Pelham. Interacting with the City of Pelham Mayor, Police Chief, Fire Chief, City Council, City Employees, and other businesses in Pelham is one of the highlights of my job. The Mayor's Executive Assistant is spearheading a bone marrow donor drive in honor of Judy. This absolutely blows us away that our community would support us in this fashion. Thankful that the faith based community continues to lift Judy towards healing. Thankful for you, our friends and family, that are joining in the chorus of prayers. Thankful for the offers to clean, cut grass, write uplifting cards and notes, food, etc, etc, etc. Thankful for Judy's Brookwood family that sent dessert goody trays to the day and night shifts at UAB Hem/Onc floor to thank them for Judy's care.

Just very very thankful. Coram DEO

5.15.2016 Update

Sunday is a day of rest, so that's what we're doing. Catnapping and then catnapping some more. Doctor Costa said this morning that they're just waiting for the white blood count to improve in order to be released home. He also said that Dr. Erba may want to start oral antibiotics and send her home anyway. He thought that the "watched pot never boils" may be the case here. Stop watching and waiting for the WBC to improve and maybe it will.

There's a song by Laura Story called 'Blessings' that has some lyrics that really speak to what I'm feeling these past few weeks:

We pray for blessings, we pray for peace. Comfort for family, protection while we sleep. We pray for healing, for prosperity. We pray for Your mighty hand to ease our suffering. All the while, You hear each spoken need. Yet love is way too much to give us lesser things. 'Cause what if Your blessings come through raindrops? What if Your healing comes through tears? What if the thousand sleepless nights are what it takes to know You're near? What if trials of this life are Your mercies in disguise?

So, we wait for His perfect timing for Judy to be able to go home. And during the wait, we see examples of His love poured out on us **every single day**. Being able to call Judy's best friend, Lisa, to stay with Judy when I can't get there till late night or early morning. Having our front flowers and bushes watered. Dogs fed. Mail gathered. Clothes washed and folded. Lawn mowed and edged. Uplifting cards sent. Telephone calls of prayer and support. Prayer and support without the telephone calls. Community thoughtfulness. Meal cards. Goody trays of thanksgiving sent to the nursing staff. Parking assistance. So much Grace in time of need. Thanks to each of you for being the hands and feet of Jesus. Coram DEO

5.16.2016 Update

So...a little bit of disappointment this morning. We were hopeful that we'd get Judy home today for a bit, however, she has been experiencing left leg pain from just below the knee down to her foot for about the past 3 days. Also her WBC is roller coastering up one day and down the next. As such, Dr. Erba wants to do some in depth testing to determine the cause. He's looking in to moving her bone marrow biopsy up from Thursday to an earlier date if possible. There is also medicine available to help boost the WBC but we need to review the trial protocol to make sure that these tests and medications are appropriate.

So...a bit of disappointment followed by a thankful and grateful heart that we have such a caring, concerned, compassionate team following her care. Continue to pray for Dr. Erba and his staff as they seek to determine these issues. Thanks! Coram DEO

5.17.2016 Update

New info just in...Dr. Erba wants to keep the original biopsy date of Thursday and possibly move it to Monday of next week. We will begin the medication today to stimulate her WBC. Her platelets are completely normal & her WBC is not, which is not how the body normally recovers from the initial chemo treatments. So...begin the WBC treatment today and see if that stimulates her body to begin making its own. We will be here for a few more days to watch the WBC.

So very thankful for a staff that is thoughtful, detailed and caring. So very thankful to be held in the palm of His hand. So very thankful He is guiding Judy's care and recovery. Coram DEO

5.19.2016 Update

So much happening in the past 2 days that I'm not really sure where to begin. So let's jump in and see where today's ramblings take us:

Thank you for the specific prayers concerning Judy's WBC. Her antibiotic was changed because the one she was on, Dr. Erba felt may be hindering her WBC recovery. The daily shot to stimulate the WBC growth was also begun. Day before yesterday her Absolute Neutrophil Count was at zero (0). Yesterday her ANC was 0.21 and this morning's labs it had climbed to 0.39. So praise to the Almighty for moving this in the correct direction. Dr. Erba also felt that if these counts improved, we may...**may**...get her home before the weekend! What a day of rejoicing that will be!

The left lower leg pain has disappeared. We don't know where it went, but we haven't gone looking for it either. Judy just received the most beautiful basket of goodies from Dr. Lawrence Lee and his staff. I was there yesterday for a medication refill and the entire staff surrounded me with questions concerning Judy. How do you properly say thank you to someone that we truly feel saved Judy's life? Words do not adequately express our thanks for the staff's knowledge, training, compassion, caring, and dedication to our health. Thank you for your continued prayers on our behalf. The gift basket contained all kinds of great snacks but the centerpiece is a beautiful cross with HOPE in the middle of it. Thanks again to Dr. Lee and staff! You've made our day.

I know I sound like a broken record (young folks...ask your parents what a record is) but we truly cannot put into words how we feel about your continued outpouring of blessings on us. Jennifer's Outlaws (Phillip's parents) and her sister-in-love took me to supper last night and we had such a sweet time of food and fellowship. Thank you again for your prayers & petitions. Coram DEO

5.20.2016 Update

This morning's post in case you missed it:

SHE'S COMING HOME TODAY!!!!!!!

All praise to Him & Him alone. More to follow when I get to my computer. This mobile update will have to do. Coram DEO

Well...it's after 18:00 on Friday evening and I've just now sat down to update the original Judy's Journey note as promised. My mobile app would not let me edit the original, hence the other brief update. Dr. Erba came in this morning and indicated her ANC had bounced way above where it needed to be in order to be released home.

I was out at Barber Motorsports Park today for the beginning of a weekend event and Lisa was more than gracious enough to get her picked up, over to Kirkland Clinic for her discharge meds, through Chick-Fil-A for lunch, and finally **HOME**. What a GREAT sound. **Home**. And guess what...she's not just home for a week or two as we had been told awhile back. She's home and doesn't have to go back in the hospital. Treatment will be continued on an outpatient basis at Kirkland Clinic! We are beyond excited, elated, blessed, ecstatic, thankful, in awe, grateful and all the other words that correlate with our feelings without breaking out the thesaurus.

Thank you to our Precious Savior that loves us more than we deserve. Thank you to the medical staffs at Lee Internal Medicine and UAB Medical Center for saving my wife. Thank you for your prayers that have certainly been, are, and will continue to be answered. Coram DEO

5.22.2016 Update

Two nights in her own bed and the dogs have not left her side. Judy's fatigue levels are still very high, but she'll do a little something and then rest for a while. She's catching up on some of her recorded shows that she missed over the past few weeks. This week we have labs on Monday with the often delayed bone marrow biopsy on Thursday. Please pray for the labs to show vast improvement as well as a rapid recovery from the biopsy. We thank you for the offers of meals and we will definitely begin taking y'all up on those when Judy's appetite returns to a more normal pallet.

Thank you for the continued prayers. They continue to be answered. Coram DEO

5.25.2016 Update

Elation & Frustration. That's where I am today if I'm being honest.

Elation because Judy's lab work from Monday looks really good to my laymen's eye. We'll find out for sure next week when we meet with Dr. Erba. But since we haven't gotten any calls from the medical team...I'm saying that's one of our small daily victories.

Frustration because I feel we obviously need to modify Judy's home medications. She is nauseated most of the time, headaches that ebb and flow, very fatigued. All things we knew that we would be facing, but now that they're staring us in the face...that's where the source of my frustration is. We'll meet with a new Nurse Practitioner tomorrow for her bone marrow biopsy and we'll see if we can get some med modification at that time. I just abhor that Judy feels so bad and there is nothing I can do to help.

I also know that the frustration comes from the father of all lies and not from Our Father that has Judy's name written in the palm of His hand. The Father that loves her and knew that we would be travelling this valley long before she was even born. Psalm 23 says that even though we walk through the valley of the shadow of death, we will fear no evil, for He is with us. I know this and I firmly believe it. I'm just being a little too human today. Coram DEO

5.27.2016 Update

Well...it's been an interesting 24 hours. As we were preparing to leave the house yesterday morning for Judy's bone marrow biopsy, she came out of the restroom and asked me "Is my eye blinking?" As she blinked, her right eyelid wasn't moving and the right side of her lip was drooping. So we sped off to the Kirkland Clinic and the lab check in lady called the stroke team. They immediately got her to the ER where a CT and an MRI were done. Stroke was ruled out however there was some indication of something going on with a narrowing of the artery in the neck area. We were admitted to the Neuro floor and this morning a CT angiogram with contrast was performed. We're waiting on the results. BTW...the bone marrow biopsy was delayed again. That's officially a bunch of times for those of you keeping score. The biopsy is again scheduled for next week but I'm not sure what the Vegas over/under is for those of you that are betting (for our non-Baptist friends). I've been trying to get the Neuro doctors to at least consult with Dr. Erba before prescribing any medications that may contraindicate what she's already on for her chemo treatment. So...please pray with us that the consultation will take place and that Judy's care will continue to be directed by the Great Physician.

I was reading this morning about Moses and his two sons as Israel was battling one of the many nations that had risen up against God's chosen people. Whenever Moses had his hands and staff in the air, Israel prevailed. When he got too tired to keep his hands in the air, his sons got him a place to sit and held his arms up for him. That is a perfect picture of the way that we feel as you come beside us and lift us up in prayer when sometimes all we can do is cry Abba, Father. Thank you for loving us. Coram DEO

5.27.2016 19:30 Update

And just like that...we're home again.

CT, MRI, Angio with contrast, and Echo, echo, echo (see what I did there?) were all negative for any stroke related issues. Thank you Jesus! The doctors have diagnosed Bell's Palsy. I've diagnosed a side effect of the Vincristine chemo drug. Either way, we've come home with a 10 day regiment of steroids. I guess I have to watch out for Judy's 'roid rage now.

The ever elusive bone marrow biopsy has been rescheduled for next Wednesday, June 1, at 1:00pm followed by the beginning of Phase 2 of her chemo induction at 2:00pm. Looks like Wednesday will be a heavy prayer request day.

Thank you, thank you, thank you for your lifting us in prayer. Each one is truly felt and appreciated. Coram DEO

5.31.2016 Update

Well, it's been a quiet few days for which we are very thankful. Judy has had 4 very restful nights in a row! Her right eyelid continues to droop and gets weary and tired towards the end of the day. Today, she has rested with her eyes closed for the majority of the day and that appears to have helped.

Tomorrow at 1:00PM is the bone marrow biopsy. She will begin phase 2 of her chemo induction at 2:00PM. As mentioned a few days ago, we covet and appreciate your prayers during these times (as well as any others that you lift us to our Lord).

Judy's appetite is slowly improving but still only takes a couple of bites and is then finished with that meal. Nausea has been very well tolerated the past few days. All in all, quiet days strung together are the little victories that we appreciate right now. But we continue to be appreciative of you, our family and friends, for the way you love us. Coram DEO

Chapter Three – June 2016

6.1.2016 Update

We're back home from the bone marrow biopsy. I wouldn't wish one of those on my worst enemy. Painful, tears, more pain, trembling, more tears and finally over. But we endure what we have to in order for Judy to get better and for others in the future that may be able to have an easier road than the one we're on.

We did not start the 2nd phase of the chemo induction this afternoon. The reasoning is that the doctor and team need the results of the biopsy to determine the next phase. Currently we are off the research trial protocol timeline because of not being able to have the biopsy performed last week due to the Bell's Palsy issue. We have a meeting next Tuesday the 7th with Dr. Erba's Nurse Practitioner to determine the next steps. Dr. Erba is the main clinical investigator for the research trial that Judy signed up for. As such, he has the ability to continue the treatment without her actually being on the study. Or...she could continue on the study as is. That is to be determined by the biopsy, lab results, and the timing parameters of the protocol.

Please pray for Judy's energy levels to drastically improve. She has absolutely no energy and her fatigue levels are maxed out. She feels like all she can do is sleep and lay on the couch or bed. The least amount of exertion just wipes her out.

We are thankful for the technology that allows us to get this message out to as many people as possible. Please feel free to share if you are led to do so. We truly appreciate the prayers of His people. Coram DEO

6.2.2016 Update

Psalm 8:9 **Oh LORD, our Lord, how majestic is your name in all the earth**.

We acknowledge that You are in complete control. You are mighty to save.

We're back in the hospital and here's what we know so far. The blood workup yesterday prior to Judy's bone marrow biopsy showed that her WBC is elevated higher than normal. The results from the biopsy are not completely back yet. What the WBC shows is that 51% are leukemia cells. As such, Dr. Erba wanted her readmitted immediately to begin an aggressive chemo regiment. I am waiting on a call from him as he was leaving immediately to catch a plane. He is to call me tonight after he gets to his destination and explain more then.

We are absolutely where we need to be. Even though we were home, she was miserable and couldn't get enough energy back to help keep her spirits up. And we know that a great attitude is necessary along with your prayers in order to fight this battle. Coram DEO

6.3.2016 Update

An aggressive chemo regiment will begin tomorrow. There will be 4 parts with an A and B phase to each. We were told to expect to stay at least another month.

So...that's what we know at this hour. I'll update more as we find out. Thank you for continuing to lift us in prayer to our Great Physician. Coram DEO

6.3.2016 – 18:00 Update
Have you ever been sitting around? Could be your office. Could be your home. Could be while you're out and about. Someone comes up to you and says "Hey! I've got good news and not so good news. Which would you like first?" Almost always we ask for the good news first. Right?

The good news is that we've surpassed our high deductible out of pocket expense for the year! The not so good news is that Judy's leukemia has returned with a vengeance.

Dr. Erba and Dr. Costa have conferred and her WBC has elevated substantially. As such, they feel that the leukemia has returned and has progressed also into her spinal column. This is evidenced by last week's Bell's Palsy episode that involved her facial nerves.

We will begin a very very aggressive regiment of chemo tomorrow with two drugs, Cytarabine and Methotrexate. Because of the high dosages of these meds, kidney damage is a possibility. They are doing some preventative meds today to assist with kidney function and are monitoring her urine output as well as uric acid levels.

Judy had a very fitful night last night. Extremely deep bone pain in her right shoulder blade area. We finally hit upon the right pain med dosage and combination this morning between 7 & 8. She has been resting comfortably since.

The other Good News that we claim is that we know Who holds and sustains Judy though this walk. He is our Great Provider. Our Great Healing Physician. Our Sustainer. The One True God. Please continue to join us in calling out to Him for strength, comfort, and total and complete healing. We love y'all! Coram DEO

6.5.2016 Update
We interrupt your Sunday afternoon nap to bring you this
news update.

The Methotrexate began late yesterday afternoon with a
high dosage flow rate for a couple of hours. The flow rate
was then reduced for the next 22 hours which we are
wrapping up by the end of this afternoon. Judy's kidneys
have been functioning correctly and her urine output
shows that the ph level is exactly where it needs to be.
Her WBC is headed in the right direction and the doctors
are pleased with her response. Later today, the
Cytarabine will begin. I think it will run for a couple of
days. So far, the chemo seems to be tolerated very well
with no pain currently and no nausea at all. She has
rested well for the past two nights and has an excellent
appetite.

We are officially off of the clinical trial that she had been
on. Because of the complications of the Bell's Palsy and
the rapid relapse of the leukemia, her doctors chose to
pursue a more aggressive therapy. With the presentation
of the Bell's Palsy, the doctors felt like one of her cranial
nerves was involved and this is one of the reasons for the
more aggressive therapies.

We are being presented with lots of risk/benefit scenarios
and the doctors are spending as much time as we need to
ask question, receive answers, consider and choose the
correct path for Judy's treatment and care. I am so
thankful that some of the world's brightest minds are
directing her care.

I am also so very thankful for a loving, praying, caring, supportive church family and friends. We truly could not make this journey on our own. Thank you to our LORD and Savior for comforting us and leading us through this.

We now return you to your regularly scheduled nap.
Coram DEO

6.6.2016 Update
Please pray the following verse with us: Isaiah 41:10 **So do not fear, for I am with you; do not be dismayed, for I am your God. I will strengthen you and help you; I will uphold you with My righteous right hand.**

72% Blast cells down to 23% down to 2%.

The Methotrexate and Cytarabine appear to be working correctly as is evidenced by the above percentages. These are the percentage of leukemia cells in Judy's blood. 72% when we arrived last Thursday. Down to 23% a couple of days ago. Now we're at the 2% level as of this morning. The goal is 0%. The Methotrexate ran for a 24 hour straight period. The Cytarabine was 4 different infusions – 1 every 12 hours. The aggressive combination of the two chemo drugs are killing off the leukemia cells and we are thankful that her other blood level numbers are looking better. We are now closely monitoring her Methotrexate level to make sure that her kidneys are flushing the meds from her system. Lots of blood work and urine analyses every few hours.

Next steps will be continued chemo through intrathecal lumbar punctures. This will place the chemo directly into Judy's spinal column. The doctors will be able to perform this procedure in her room at the bedside.

Judy has been sleeping for most of yesterday and today. We're thankful for no pain so she can catch up on some much needed rest. Please pray that her energy levels will increase where we can start to cruise the hallways again. Coram DEO

6.8.2016 Update

Tomorrow Judy will have chemo through intrathecal lumbar puncture. This will place the chemo directly into her spinal column. Doctors will be able to perform this procedure in her room at the bedside. She has to lay flat on her back for at least an hour after the procedure in order to minimize the possibility of a spinal headache. The good thing about having it done at the bedside vs the clinic is the staff is able to give a sedative to aid in pain relief and relaxation.

Judy has been awake for most of today. We're thankful for no pain so she can catch up on some much needed rest. She has, however, been dealing with the sour stomach and had diarrhea all last night. She is currently on contact precautions (gown, gloves & mask) for anyone coming in the room. A stool sample was sent to the lab this morning for testing but we haven't gotten results back yet. The doctors feel it is chemo induced but want to make sure it isn't some type of infection.

We are asked all the time "What can we do?" Pray. And then pray some more. Our yard is being taken care of. Our dogs are being looked after. Kat Baglini (one of our daughter's best friends) and Wendy Ainsworth (my boss) set up the You Caring site to help defray expenses that we incur. Currently that is mostly parking, outside meals from the food court and surrounding restaurants for Rick, and the co-pays that are starting to come in from insurance. I promise it won't go towards a beach vacation when we blow this Popsicle stand!

I know I say this all the time but we really do thank you for your prayers. We feel them. God hears them. He acts on them. May He receive all the glory due His Holy Name for the healing He is bringing about. We love y'all. Coram DEO

6.10.2016 Update
Yesterday, as you know, Judy had chemo through intrathecal lumbar puncture. The doctors were able to perform this procedure in her room at the bedside. We haven't gotten the full report back yet but, the preliminary report shows that the spinal fluid is clear of any leukemia. She had no spinal headache from the procedure and has tolerated the chemo very well.

The sour stomach continues to hang around and the diarrhea has diminished but continues as well. The stool sample came back negative for an infection so the contact precautions have been removed. They are really pushing fluids via IV today to prevent dehydration from the constant bathroom runs. The pharmacy is brewing a cocktail to aid in settling Judy's stomach down. She'll receive that later today.

That's all we know at this time. We're on a monitor the blood work timeline. Based on what the doctors' review from the blood work, they determine next steps. That's the hardest portion of what we're facing. The uncertainty of next steps. But we rely on the One who is under control of His timeframe. We simply have to trust His timing and His direction of Judy's medical team. We love y'all. Coram DEO

6.12.2016 Update
Sunday afternoon. Quiet. Peaceful. Relaxing. Refreshing.
A time of renewal. Great naps.

Judy has had two GREAT nights in a row of restful sleep
with no pain, nausea, or diarrhea. Her appetite is slowly
returning and the food is settling with no tummy
rumbles! Thank you LORD for the relief and rest that
only comes from You.

During rounds this morning, Dr. Costa said we are in the
wait, test, review, and monitor phase. She will receive the
shots again to kick start her WBC. They are so good at
watching the blood test results and determining the next
steps. It's a fine line of balancing between killing the
leukemia and killing it too quickly. If they kill the
leukemia too quickly, we run the risk of damaging Judy's
bone marrow as well as damage internal organs and then
we're looking at a whole different ballgame. We're very
thankful for the superior intelligence of the entire
medical team directing Judy's care.

I will head back to work tomorrow as I've been at the
hospital with Judy since being readmitted. I'm so grateful
to work for a company that understands. Pray that I can
focus on work things when I need to focus on work
things. Because Judy's care is being directed by the Best
Hands possible. Thank you LORD for Judy's care. May
we always give You the glory and honor due Your Name.
Coram DEO

6.15.2016 Update
Judy has had several GREAT nights in a row of restful sleep with no pain or nausea. She's currently sitting beside me on the couch eating a chocolate Mighty Shake!

We are still in the wait, test, review, and monitor phase. She is receiving the Granix injections to help kick start her WBC. She developed a fever two nights ago that the staff said they were actually waiting to happen. With her immune system basically wiped out, even the smallest of infections can develop from things that are normally routine in nature and occur on skin anyway. They've run 4 blood cultures and 2 of the 4 have already come back positive. The other 2 are still 'cooking' and will be in over the next couple of days. Judy has been receiving 2 different broad spectrum antibiotics and the fever broke around 3:00AM night before last.

Our church has a Bible reading application that you can read on a daily basis or it will read it to you! Yesterday's scripture was Philippians 1. Verses 12 through 26 are an excellent example to me of how Judy is approaching this leukemia diagnosis. Her faith is truly amazing and is a joy to see in her suffering. Glory to God. Coram DEO

6.19.2016
Happy Father's Day from UAB Hospital!

Today is the day that the LORD has made. We will
rejoice and be glad in it. We especially rejoice this
Father's Day because we found out this morning that
Judy will possibly be released to go home this Tuesday!!!
Happy Father's Day to me!!! We are so excited to get her
home again. The plan is to have another bone marrow
biopsy in another week and review with Dr. Erba when
the results are back. Then we'll know what our next steps
are.

Please pray that Judy will not have any fear about the
leukemia returning again. She was tearful with the doctor
this morning during rounds and her biggest concern is
that we won't be a loop of kill it and it comes back, kill it
and it comes back. We know that God is in complete
control of the outcome. Our fervent prayer is that our
faith won't be overshadowed by our fear. Fear has been
defined as False Expectations Appearing Real. Another
definition that I've found is Face Everything And
Rejoice. I like that one a lot more and that's the one
we're claiming.

Thank you for the way you continue to lift us and love
us. It is truly humbling to see His people in action.
Coram DEO

6.21.2016 Update

Hello Tuesday! It's good to see you! Especially with Judy home from the hospital and sleeping in her own bed!! Maggie on one side and Belle on the other. (Belle replaced me when I got up). They sure were happy to see her get out of the truck yesterday. I wonder why they don't get that excited to see me?

Judy was released a day earlier than expected due to her blood levels rapidly coming back into safe range. This was what was keeping her in the hospital that 5th week of the first stay, waiting on her levels to recover from the chemo wiping everything out. Her body is responding positively on its own this time. Praise Him!

A home health agency is coming to the house today to teach us home infusion. Judy was receiving a 14 day regiment of antibiotic and was 8 days into the treatment. She'll have another 6 IV infusions here at home. This is due to two of the 4 blood cultures showing positive for bacterial growth. I feel like I need to go stay at a Holiday Inn Express so I'll have the correct medical knowledge to treat her properly. Thankfully, we have much wiser and knowledgeable people guiding us. I've tried to stay away from Google and WebMD. Those sites can have you running for the hills.

So…on to What's Next? Judy will continue home infusion therapy for the next 6 days. We have an 8:30AM appointment next Thursday the 30th at Kirkland Clinic for a bone marrow biopsy with labs at 7:30AM. We will discuss the results with Dr. Erba at her 4:00PM appointment on July 6th. Our hospital discharge notes tell us to be prepared to be readmitted for chemo treatment. This is not a shock or unexpected. Before we were discharged yesterday, the Nurse Practitioner said that future chemo treatments would be done inpatient rather than in clinic. We are not expecting to have lengthy stays with these treatments.

Y'all…it is hard for me to explain how much I love this woman. She is absolutely the definition of grace under fire. As escort came to get us yesterday, nurses and patient care technicians were coming out of rooms and hallways to say goodbye. Judy has invested as much in them as they have in her. She cares about their families, their career paths, and most of all…their souls. Even in the midst of this leukemia trial, Judy has never lost hope in the One Who sustains. The One Who gives everlasting life. The One True Hope. It is her heartfelt fervent prayer that others come to this knowledge, love, and hope.
Coram DEO

6.29.2016 Update
Hey Y'all!! Remember us?

Judy has been at home recuperating now for several days. She's still as weak as a kitten but we see small improvements each and every day. Her appetite ebbs and flows with the amount of stomach sourness during each day. But we see that improving each day as well. She is sleeping very well at night and has been able to stay awake during the day. She's been catching up on her recorded TV programs and has been able to concentrate on them. Small daily victories.

Amedisys Home Health agency came to the house to teach us how to do home infusion. Judy received 6 IV antibiotic infusions. This was due to two of the 4 blood cultures showing positive for bacterial growth while she was in-patient. She was tested for C-Diff here at home as well which came back negative and we are grateful for that result.

We have an 8:30AM appointment tomorrow the 30th at Kirkland Clinic for a bone marrow biopsy with labs at 7:30AM. I spoke with the clinic today to ask if pain medication was available for Judy as the first bone marrow biopsy was horrid. She will have meds available to relax her as well as pain management. We will discuss the results with Dr. Erba at Judy's 4:00PM appointment on July 6th. I received a call from UAB Admitting today and Judy will be readmitted on the 6th for chemo treatment. This is not a shock or unexpected. We are not expecting to have lengthy stays with these treatments.

We continue to be humbled by the outpouring of love and concern for us. Please continue your prayers for Judy's comfort, strength, and healing. Coram DEO

6.30.2016

When God hears His people's prayers of petition for one of His children, WOW does He answer and bring glory to Himself.

Judy's bone marrow biopsy could not have been any more different this time over last time. To quote Judy when her Nurse Practitioner was finished with the procedure – "That's it?" Not a whimper. Not a shriek. No tears (other than tears of happiness and thanksgiving). Minimal discomfort. NO PAIN. Thank you LORD for hearing our prayers.

The NP went over the lab results from this morning and they were all very close to being in normal ranges across the board. Her body is responding to the treatments much better this round. We'll start chemo again next Wednesday after the visit with Dr. Erba.

As we were leaving the clinic, I asked Judy if she wanted to run through somewhere and get food to take home and she said "No. I want to go to McAlister's and sit there for lunch". This was her first outing since April that didn't involve the hospital or clinic.

Thank you for your prayers on Judy's behalf. She approached this BMB with very little anxiety considering what she went through the first time. To God be the glory, great things He has done. Coram DEO

Chapter Four – July 2016

7.1.2016
July. New month. New challenges.

Dr. Erba just called with the preliminary results from Judy's bone marrow biopsy from yesterday afternoon. There is just no other way to say it. The leukemia is still present. Dr. Erba said that it is not as prevalent as previous results as are indicated by her White Blood Count being close to normal parameters but, it is still there.

Judy will be readmitted to UAB tomorrow to begin treatment with the medication that she would have received if she had remained on the clinical trial. It is a 28 day infusion period for which she will be in-patient for the first few days and released home for the remainder of the infusion period.

Dr. Erba indicated that he had some other therapies that he has been developing that he wants to talk to us about tomorrow as well. Insurance has denied these new therapies; however, Dr. Erba said he will educate the insurance folks on leukemia treatments. I'm so very thankful for this man's insight and intelligence.

So…New month…New challenges. But these challenges are absolutely no surprise what so ever to our God. He knew before Judy was created that she would be walking this path. We are thankful the He is the Lamp for our feet and the Light for our path. We just need to stay the course.

Thank you that you will continue to lift us in prayer to our Creator and our Savior. We truly appreciate y'all. Coram DEO

7.3.2016

Random thoughts from this morning's visit with Dr.
Erba: Blincyto, targeted gene therapy, cytokine release
syndrome (CRS), CD19 chromosome, CD3 chromosome,
two defective genes within chromosomes causing the
leukemia cells to receive messages to constantly
replicate, DNA, Jakafi (Jak2 inhibitor), binding,
explanation of why the first two chemo rounds didn't put
Judy into remission, side effects, 28 day constant
infusion, insurance acceptance, insurance denial, rarity,
enzymes talking to cell nuclei, chaining, Step C, Step D.
Wow. We have a lot to process.

The reason that the first two chemo treatments (Steps A
& B) didn't put Judy into remission is because of the
rarity of what is happening on the cellular & molecular
levels in her body. As we understand what Dr. Erba was
explaining, Judy has within her DNA one defective
chromosome that has genes that have bound together
sending messages to the cell nuclei to constantly replicate
the leukemia cells. The therapy (Step D) that Dr. Erba
wanted to discuss with us that will possibly be the best
route is actually the one the insurance company is
denying because her specific type and subtype of
leukemia is not listed on the Jakafi drug therapy cancer
types. This is what Dr. Erba was saying he was going to
have to educate the insurance company on cancer
therapies and treatments.

Judy will begin the Blincyto therapy (Step C) this
afternoon around 3:00. This therapy is the one that Judy
would have received if she had remained on the clinical
trial. This is the 28 day constant infusion that can have

the main side effects of fever, chills, and aches. Blincyto therapy can also cause cytokine release syndrome which will be closely monitored throughout the infusion. This is not chemotherapy but an antibody therapy that causes Judy's body to react as if she were fighting an infection.

With that mouthful being said, we continue to appreciate your prayers on Judy's behalf. We still have a very long road in front of us; however, at least we know why the first two standard chemo rounds weren't effective and we have a game plan mapped out. Please pray for the insurance company to clearly understand the therapy that Dr. Erba has mapped out and to approve it. Pray for minimal to zero side effects from the Blincyto therapy. Pray that through Judy's Journey that others will clearly have an easier path to follow. To God be the glory. Coram DEO

7.8.2016

Judy began the Blincyto 28 day antibody therapy Sunday afternoon around 4:00. As expected, the main side effects of fever, chills, and nausea reared their heads beginning around 8:30 Sunday night. Fevers gradually rose to 102 throughout the night with chills setting in Monday morning. A brief bout of nausea hit around mid-afternoon. A course of steroids and antibiotics were started and she was able to sleep peacefully through the beautiful Thunder on the Mountain fireworks display Monday night. The fever and chills abated Monday evening and Judy has had excellent days Tuesday and Wednesday. For the first 24 to 48 hours of infusion, Judy's vital signs were taken every 2 hours and monitored extremely close. This was because the Blincyto therapy can also cause cytokine release syndrome (CRS) which can have dire consequences if not closely monitored throughout the infusion. CRS is a common immediate complication occurring with the use of anti-T cell antibody infusions which is what the Blincyto treatment falls into. CRS is not what my Dad use to say as he got older. His definition was Can't Remember S%&@. Sure do miss him.

Our social worker, Molly, has begun the task of talking with insurance to determine if we can continue the infusion at home or if we have to stay in-patient for the whole 28 day period. We should hear something concerning that very soon. Whether it's a go home or stay in-patient decision, we pray that whichever is the best direction for Judy's safety is the one that bubbles to the surface. After the 28 days is completed, we will have a 2 week rest period. At the end of the 2 weeks, Judy will have another bone marrow biopsy to see where we stand.

I'm so very thankful that the infusion reaction was as short a time period as it was. I'm thankful for a medical staff that checked on her throughout that first 24 hour period. I'm thankful for a church family that supports us through visits and prayers. I'm thankful for technology that allows our story to reach you. I'm thankful for Judy's sweet spirit and her "I'll beat this" attitude. I'm thankful for a merciful God that hears our every prayer. I'm thankful for a merciful God that hears my groaning when words don't come. I'm thankful for a community that thinks enough of our family to hold fund raisers in our honor.

Mostly, I'm thankful that y'all read my ramblings and pray for my precious Judy. To God be the glory. Coram DEO

7.9.2016
We made it to the weekend! Welcome to Saturday everyone!

Since the initial reaction to the Blincyto treatment that was started last Sunday, Judy has had progressively better and better days throughout the week. Dr. Erba is extremely pleased with her reaction to the treatment. Each day we've seen increased appetite, less sour stomach, better blood work, and more wanting to do things on her own. Yesterday (Friday) was the best day yet with great appetite and no sour stomach for the entire day! The current plan is to complete this 28 day infusion cycle. We will have a two week resting period followed by another bone marrow biopsy to determine the initial Blincyto treatment results. Another 28 day Blincyto infusion will then be initiated. After the second cycle, discussions are underway for a bone marrow transplant.

We have several things we're working on that need your prayers please. The staff is working with insurance to determine if we can complete the Blincyto treatment at home rather than remain in-patient. The dosage is scheduled to be increased tomorrow afternoon. Whether we remain in-patient or are released home, our prayer is that we are in the safest place for Judy considering the possible side effects of the treatment. The next prayer request is a huge one (but never to huge for our God to knock down to manageable size). Currently, the insurance company (Blue Cross Blue Shield of Texas) is saying that the In Network, Tenet Preferred Transplant Centers are in Long Island, New York or in Colorado. While the thought of seeing if Billy Joel would welcome us into his Long Island estate for an extended stay, we'd really rather stay right here at UAB. We're 12 miles from home. Our family, church and community support systems are right here and highly supportive and effective. Judy is currently under treatment right here. All her testing has been done right here. It just makes sense to have everything done right here. There are a plethora of pre-transplant procedures that have to be done in a timely fashion and with Judy still under extensive treatment, it just makes sense to continue right here.

I've said right here a bunch in the previous paragraph. Right here is where God lead us 24 years ago. Right here is where our children were raised. Right here is family. Right here is community. Right here is our church family. We want to see Judy healed…Right Here. Thank you for joining us in prayer. We are humbled that you lead us into His throne room each and every day. We love y'all. Coram DEO

7.12.2016 Update

Zip, zilch, nada, zero, diddly, zippo, goose egg, nary. These are the official medical descriptions of Judy's side effects from the Blincyto dosage increase on Sunday afternoon! No fever. No chills. No nausea. We're very thankful that the reaction to the increased dosage was tolerated as well as can be expected. Thank you Lord! We're still waiting to hear from insurance to determine if we can complete the Blincyto treatment at home rather than remain in-patient. Dr. Erba feels like we should be able to be home by the weekend.

I had discussions with the insurance company (Blue Cross Blue Shield of Texas) yesterday concerning the Transplant Centers in New York or Colorado as well as with Tenet Advocacy Services. Tenet (owner of Brookwood Hospital) is self-insured and BCBS of TX is the administrator of the policy. Any changes, exemptions, or exceptions to the policy have to be determined and approved through Tenet. Tenet's Advocacy Services is supposed to get back with me no later than the 18th with a decision. This is the decision that we pray allows Judy to remain right here at UAB for the proposed bone marrow transplant. There is so much pre-testing, typing, and donor matching that must take place prior to the transplant. We also pray that it will be considered In-Network and Tenet Preferred as far as claims payment is concerned.

Y'all continue to amaze us with your generosity. The get well cards, gift cards, gift bags, text messages, goody bags, phone calls, and prayers lift our spirits and make us

truly thankful for your friendship. We are truly humbled.
Coram DEO

7.15.2016 Update
Sing with us:

Praise to the Lord, the Almighty, the King of creation!
O my soul, praise Him, for He is thy health and salvation!
All ye who hear, now to His temple draw near;
praise Him in glad adoration.

There is quite a lot to update our friends and prayer warriors on for this week's happenings. Judy did experience about 48 hours of increased fevers beginning early Wednesday morning from the Blincyto therapy. The doctors feel like it is a normal side effect and are not overly concerned. They ran blood cultures as a precaution and those have come back negative so far. The infusion company is in discussion with insurance to see what type of reimbursement will be covered if Judy is allowed to go home to continue the infusion. We should have a decision somewhere around the 18th. So…for the time being, we're still at UAB.

Now for the phenomenal news of the week; after several discussions with Blue Cross Blue Shield of Texas Customer Service, Blue Cross Blue Shield Transplant Case Manager, Tenet Advocacy Services, UAB Transplant Center and our Nurse Practitioners, we will be allowed to remain Right Here at UAB for the bone marrow transplant!!! Let me say that again…we will be allowed to remain Right Here at UAB for the bone marrow transplant!!! And because we have satisfied our out of pocket maximum for the year, all transplant related expenses will be 100% covered. Praise the LORD!

Folks, this phenomenal news has been brought to you by your prayers. How can we begin to say thank you? How do we begin to express our gratitude? The only way we know is to include you in our prayers of thanks to Him Who is able. A simple thank you just sounds hollow but, that's what we offer to Him Who hears. Thank you. Coram DEO

7.19.2016 Update
And the hits just keep on coming!!!!!!!

Blincyto home infusion approved!
Meeting with home infusion specialist completed!
Bone Marrow Transplant officially certified for
Birmingham!
Meeting with BMT Transplant Coordinator completed!
Initial BMT testing and typing completed on Judy!
Typing kits prepped for Judy's brother & sister!
My sister is coming this Saturday for a visit!
Our God is still very much on His throne!!!!!!!

Coram DEO

7.22.2016 Update
Happy Friday Everyone! Welcome to summer in the
South.

Judy was released home on Wednesday to continue her
Blincyto treatment. Two restful nights sleeping in her
own bed have been remarkable. The dogs were ecstatic to
see her and have not left her side. I was pretty excited to
get her home as well.

Coram CVS is the supplier of the medication for Judy's
home infusion and they came early Wednesday afternoon
to train us on the infusion pump and how to change the
medication bags. Each bag runs for 48 hours and we
change bags every two days. The pump and medication
fit into a fanny pack looking bag so Judy isn't connected
to an IV pole. This creates a situation where we have to
keep a closer eye on Judy so she doesn't bolt and run! As
our Pastor says…Oh Hah!

Before we were discharged Wednesday, one of our
nurses stopped by to say goodbye to Judy and prayed
Psalm 71:14 over Judy:

> ***But as for me, I will always have hope;***
> ***I will praise you more and more.***

She said that verse really reminded her of Judy because
she displays hope in every situation that she's faced. To
me, that's one of the greatest compliments that can be
paid to someone. That Jesus our Hope, shines through in
every situation we face.

So what's next? We have our first bag change this afternoon around 3:00. We go for labs on Monday the 25th and August 1st. Bone marrow biopsy on the 8th with doctor visit and results on the 15th. We expect to have another round of Blincyto at that point. A bone marrow transplant is in the works. Judy's brother has had labs drawn to determine if he is a match. Judy's sister was supposed to receive her kit this week as well. With no offence intended to Judy's sister, we hoping that her brother will be the match as it will be easier for all if donor and patient are in close proximity due to the intensive procedure of testing, matching, and transplant. If neither brother nor sister is a match, then the national database will be searched. If no match is still found, Matt & Jennifer will be tested.

So there you have pretty much everything we know at this point. We love and appreciate your prayers. They truly are felt. Coram DEO

7.27.2016 Update

My Great-Great Grandfather was a Scottish sea Captain named Alexander Sim whom my middle name comes from. His ship was a barque (sailing vessel with three or more masts) named the Palestine. His textile and cattle trade route was between England and Australia. I've grown up around water and have been sailing since the age of 7. In addition to dreaming of being a cowboy or astronaut when growing up, I also fancied having a touch of pirate blood as well. I'm currently reading a series of books in which the main character traces his heritage back to Blackhawke, the famous pirate. In the current book there is a line that really struck a chord with me this week:

I imagine our marriage will be a sturdy little barque upon which to ride out the tumult.

Tumult is certainly an emotion that we could have turned to when we heard the news: *Judy has leukemia.* To say our world was turned upside down would be an understatement. Instead of tumult, we chose to turn to our Lord and Saviour to guide us through this journey, just as He has always done. He has lit and smoothed our path each and every step and already has the result in hand.

This past Monday we had a blood workup for Judy and the results were very good. Her hematocrit and hemoglobin were higher than they've been in three months. In the lab waiting room, she was able to meet a gentleman that is about a year ahead of Judy in the same treatment regimen. They were able to talk about their shared experiences and I think it was really helpful for

her. We'll have another blood workup this coming
Monday with the bone marrow biopsy the following
Monday.

Thank you for the continued prayers on our behalf. We
love y'all. Coram DEO

Chapter Five – August 2016

8.6.2016 Update

This past Monday, August 1st, we had another blood workup for Judy and the results were even better than the previous Monday. The first Blincyto treatment was completed on Sunday afternoon and Judy has been infusion pump free all week! Her energy levels continue to improve each day with added strength and stamina. On the way home from the blood workup on Monday she said she wanted to go shopping which should put fear into any husband's heart, but it absolutely thrilled me. We stopped at Publix and put Judy in one of the motorized Granny Carts and turned her loose. She didn't knock over any displays and I came out of the grocery store with all 10 toes still intact.

This coming Monday, the 8th, we will go in for a bone marrow biopsy which will determine our next steps and give us a better view into what the antibody treatment accomplished. Our goal is to be able to go the entire week without hearing from Dr. Erba until our appointment with him on the 15th. To date we've always heard from him the following day after the biopsy telling us to come back in for admission to the hospital.

We aren't really sure of next steps until after the doctor visit, but we'll have a clearer picture then. We're hopeful and prayerful that we'll hear that Judy is in remission at that point. Past that, it could be another round of Blincyto. Could be she is presented for a bone marrow transplant. We don't really know but we are relying on the One that has guided us thus far. He knows and will reveal it in His timing, not ours.

We are so very thankful for technology and for the medical advancements God has revealed that have allowed Judy to progress this far. Without the Blincyto treatment, we don't really know where we would be since the chemo treatments didn't work for her. But all praise to Him Who is able. As always…thanks to you for the continued prayers on our behalf. We love y'all.
Coram DEO

8.13.2016 Update
This past Monday, the 8th, we had the bone marrow biopsy and the nurse practitioner called today saying the results are normal. Let me repeat…NORMAL!!! Judy asked if this meant the Blincyto was working and she said that's exactly what it means. All praise to Him Who is able! We will have another lumbar puncture tomorrow morning so that all results will be available for our Dr. Erba visit on Monday the 15th. We have not heard the word 'remission' yet, but we remain hopeful that we'll heard that beautiful word this coming Monday.

Judy woke up Monday morning with double vision. We've been to the Eye Foundation Hospital for a total eye workup as well as an MRI. The MRI has come back as normal so, we're waiting to hear if this could be a side effect of one of the treatments she's had.

We also met with the transplant coordinator on Monday and Judy has match options in the national databank. We still aren't really sure of next steps until after the doctor visit, but we'll have a clearer picture then. We're still hopeful and prayerful that we'll hear that Judy is in remission at that point. Past that, it could be another round of Blincyto. Could be she is presented for the bone marrow transplant. We don't really know but we are relying on the One that has guided us thus far. He knows and will reveal it in His timing, not ours.

Thank You God for these little victories. Please continue to guide us and direct us. We completely rely on You. Coram DEO

8.15.2016 Update

Exactly four months ago today, April the 15th, we heard the dreadful words…Judy, you have leukemia. Little did we realize the journey that we were about to embark upon. But that journey has led us to today, August the 15th, where we heard the beautiful words…Judy, you're in remission. That's right…REMISSION!!!!!!! Tears of joy along with quiet prayers of thanks and gratitude filled the remainder of the afternoon and evening. Thank You LORD for Your favor upon Judy and her phenomenal care team.

Judy was readmitted late this afternoon to the UAB Hematology/Oncology floor for the beginning of the second treatment of Blincyto. Dr. Erba wants to delay the treatment a couple of days in order to run some extensive tests on Judy to determine what is going on with her eyes, the double vision, and headaches. The double vision in the right eye seems to have diminished, however it has migrated to her left eye now. Dr. Erba wants to have a Neuro-Ophthalmologist run some tests along with additional lumbar punctures just to make sure that the leukemia isn't hiding in her ocular nerves. Even though the LP from Thursday was clear of any leukemia cells, it will take a few more lumbar punctures just to make sure. He does not feel that it is a side effect of the Blincyto treatment.

We also met with the transplant coordinator and one of the transplant doctors today as well. Judy does have matches in the national databank and the process is moving forward to have the additional testing done on the potential donors.

Thank You God for these huge victories. It is by Your hand that we are where we are. Please continue to lift Judy up in prayer. As you can tell…they are definitely heard. Coram DEO

8.19.2016 Update
Greetings from the 7th floor of UAB hospital on this rainy Friday evening!

Judy had a bunch of tests done this week and Dr. Erba just met with us to discuss all the results and a plan to move forward. The lumbar puncture performed on Tuesday did indicate that there is a minute trace of leukemia cells (0.36%) that are involving the cranial nerves dealing with her eyes and sight. This was the cause of the double vision and the migration of symptoms from the right eye to the left. Another LP with intrathecal chemo cocktail was performed this afternoon to help with the hiding leukemia cells. The Blincyto was successful as far as the leukemia in the blood and bone marrow. It will not cross the blood/brain barrier hence the reasoning behind the thought process to move forward with radiation of the cranial nerves. After the Blincyto, Judy will go through whole body radiation and high dose chemo anyway in preparation for the bone marrow transplant so Dr. Erba felt this was the logic next step. We'll probably meet with the radiation doctors on Monday and will develop a plan for outpatient treatment.

We would appreciate your prayers for God's continued guidance of Dr. Erba and all of the consulting doctors. The knowledge and compassion they display on a daily basis is amazing. Thank you for your prayers for Judy. We love y'all. Coram DEO

8.21.2016 Update

We have a new treatment that will be our newest mouthful to say and try to understand: Craniospinal Irradiation. It's just the fancy way to say that she's gonna get nuked in her brain and spine. BTW…cancer sucks. The lumbar puncture on Friday confirmed the presence of a minute trace of leukemia cells in her Cranial Spinal Fluid (CSF). Judy was taken downstairs this morning for a CT in preparation for her radiation treatment. This CT was to map out the head and spine areas as well as create a facial mask that will be utilized for the radiation. She said the mask was very claustrophobic until she relaxed and realized it's porous and she could actually breathe! BTW…cancer sucks. We will have a two part MRI that could begin this evening or early tomorrow morning to also assist in preparation. The radiation is scheduled for 1:00PM tomorrow afternoon.

So tomorrow will be a very packed day. MRI, radiation, Blincyto bag change, and whatever else may be presented. BTW…cancer sucks. Please pray for Judy's stamina as she is very tired from having severe headaches the past few days. Nausea has also reared its ugly head yesterday and today. She is currently knocked out with some Phenergan.

I don't know if you know this or not but…cancer sucks. Thank you for the way that you continually love on us. We so appreciate the calls, cards, and prayers. We love y'all. Coram DEO

8.30.2016

I'd like to share some information with you today, the 35th anniversary of my 27th birthday. Cancer still sucks. But the good news that we can share with you today is Judy's last two CTs have come back negative for blast cells after running the flow cytometry. What a fantastic birthday present to hear that all the treatments are working. Thank you God for Your favor!

The Craniospinal Irradiation continues and Judy has completed 4 of 12 treatments. Her vision continues to improve as well. Please pray for her strength and stamina. She is just exhausted from the last 2 weeks in-patient. We got home yesterday and had a pretty good first night; however, she's got some sleep to catch up on.

This update is short and sweet but none the less heartfelt in my appreciation for your prayers on our behalf. They are truly felt.

2 Corinthians 4:16-18

Therefore we do not lose heart. Though outwardly we are wasting away, yet inwardly we are being renewed day by day. For our light and momentary troubles are achieving for us an eternal glory that far outweighs them all. So we fix our eyes not on what is seen, but on what is unseen, since what is seen is temporary, but what is unseen is eternal.

Coram DEO

Chapter Six – September 2016

9.5.2016

Happy Non-Labor Day to us! We've had three glorious days at home with no sticks, no punctures, no radiation treatments, no appetite, no 4:00AM blood draws, no appointments, nowhere we had to be other than resting right here.

The Craniospinal Irradiation will continue Tuesday through Friday and Judy has completed 7 of 12 treatments with the final treatment next Monday. Only 5 more to go! Please pray for her anxiety level to greatly reduce as she really doesn't like the radiation treatments. Each treatment has increased in length and being held down on the table by the radiation mask really gets to her towards the end of treatment time.

The last three lumbar punctures have come back negative for blast cells in the cranial spinal fluid which means they have been reduced to only once per week. Her double vision has cleared up as well.

We are continually blown away with the way God is moving in Judy's care. The timing of appointments, treatments, travel, cards & letters, calls, and the list could go on and on. His perfect timing is clearly evident in every step of our journey. To Him be glory and praise.

2 Corinthians 4:16-18

Therefore we do not lose heart. Though outwardly we are wasting away, yet inwardly we are being renewed day by day. For our light and momentary troubles are achieving for us an eternal glory that far

outweighs them all. So we fix our eyes not on what is seen, but on what is unseen, since what is seen is temporary, but what is unseen is eternal.

Coram DEO

9.6.2016 Update

Well…just like that, we're back in the hospital. We went in today for the radiation treatment and her blood work showed decreased counts across the board. She's also a touch dehydrated so Judy has been readmitted.

On a happy note…the radiation treatment went very well today. The session only lasted 30 minutes today which Judy handles very well. It's the sessions that go closer to 45 minutes to an hour that are the ones that are really tough for her. Only 4 more sessions to go! Thanks for the continued prayer!

2 Corinthians 4:16-18

Therefore we do not lose heart. Though outwardly we are wasting away, yet inwardly we are being renewed day by day. For our light and momentary troubles are achieving for us an eternal glory that far outweighs them all. So we fix our eyes not on what is seen, but on what is unseen, since what is seen is temporary, but what is unseen is eternal.

Coram DEO

9.11.2016
On this day when we remember the 2001 attacks on our great nation, please remember our first responders that continue to stand in the gap to keep us safe each and every day. The men and women that run to the fight rather than away.
John 15:13 **Greater love has no one than this: to lay down one's life for one's friends.**

Judy was released late yesterday and had a great first night back at home. We received absolutely fantastic news as well. Based on 4 negative flow reports from the lumbar punctures, Judy has been declared in remission. No evidence of leukemia blast cells in her blood, marrow, cerebral spinal fluid, or cranial nerves. To God be the glory, great things He has done.

We meet with Dr. Erba tomorrow for a checkup and will hopefully find out a timeline for transplant. Tomorrow is also her last radiation treatment (Yea!!!) and we will meet with Dr. Marcus Bredel (her Radiation Oncologist) to review all her scans. Thursday will be her final Blincyto infusion as well. So…big week ahead with lots of anticipated answers.

2 Corinthians 4:16-18
Therefore we do not lose heart. Though outwardly we are wasting away, yet inwardly we are being renewed day by day. For our light and momentary troubles are achieving for us an eternal glory that far outweighs them all. So we fix our eyes not on what is

seen, but on what is unseen, since what is seen is temporary, but what is unseen is eternal.

Thank you for the continued prayers on our behalf. We love y'all. Coram DEO

9.16.2016 Update

Yesterday was the 5 month anniversary of Judy's Journey. What a ride it has been thus far. Since the new episodes of various TV shows will be starting in the next few weeks, I thought we'd begin this update like this:

Previously on Judy's Journey:

This past Monday we were supposed to meet with Dr. Erba for an office visit, however, Judy decided she wanted an ambulance ride instead to the emergency room. As we were getting ready to leave for the doctor appointment, her speech became garbled and she was trying to repeat the same phrase which was coming out jumbled and garbled. I called 911 and Engine 94 & paramedics from the Pelham Fire Department rapidly arrived. They assessed her and an ambulance ride to UAB ensued. Judy was readmitted to the Hem/Onc floor later that day and was placed in the Judy McCoy Memorial Room 7352. Somehow she got back into the same room we were just released from last week. The incredible staff on the 7th floor said that rarely happens. After much poking, prodding, CT, blood cultures, etc, etc, etc, Dr. Erba determined that the garbled speech was a side effect of the Blincyto. This side effect typically presents during the first week of the first infusion but Judy likes to do things a little differently!

Final radiation treatment was completed on Wednesday with the final Blincyto infusion of round 2 completed yesterday. We were released home early yesterday evening and we're going to try and make a normal doctor appointment on Monday.

Thank you to our incredible church family for the way y'all have checked on us, prayed with us, loved us through this journey. It really is the people and not the building.

2 Corinthians 4:16-18
Therefore we do not lose heart. Though outwardly we are wasting away, yet inwardly we are being renewed day by day. For our light and momentary troubles are achieving for us an eternal glory that far outweighs them all. So we fix our eyes not on what is seen, but on what is unseen, since what is seen is temporary, but what is unseen is eternal.

Thank you for the continued prayers on our behalf. We love y'all. Coram DEO

9.23.2016 Update

This past Monday we were to meet with Dr. Erba for an office visit, however, he wanted Judy to have another bone marrow biopsy before he saw her again. So, Tuesday afternoon, she had one. On Wednesday, she had another lumbar puncture (LP). We'll meet with Dr. Erba next Wednesday the 28th to discuss the results. I suggested to Judy that we should go to the courthouse and change her middle name to Pincushion. This was the 5th bone marrow biopsy and the 13th LP since April.

After 5 long months of this journey, we now have a tentative date for the bone marrow transplant which is October 25th. From the beginning of the month until the 25th, Ole Pincushion, I mean Judy, will have a stem to stern workup to include pulmonary testing, x-ray, cardiac tests of EKG & Echo, consultations, lumbar puncture, port placement, total body irradiation and a partridge in a pear tree.

As you can see, we still have a very long road in front of us. Please pray for Judy's stamina, increased appetite, decreased to nonexistent nausea, no neurological issues, toleration of the pre-transplant medications, and especially for the 23 year old young gentleman that is Judy's donor. Without his selfless donation, Judy's outcome would be bleak indeed.

Please also pray for a huge turnout for a bone marrow drive in Judy's honor on October 13th at the Pelham Civic Center and Ice Arena from 3:00PM until 7:00PM. The City of Pelham is hosting this event with Be The Match Registry and we are truly humbled for their love for us.

It's simply a cheek swab and fill out some paperwork. It couldn't be simpler. Our donor took the time and effort to participate in a drive in the past and we can't wait to thank him for saving Judy's life. Please participate. Thanks!

2 Corinthians 4:16-18

Therefore we do not lose heart. Though outwardly we are wasting away, yet inwardly we are being renewed day by day. For our light and momentary troubles are achieving for us an eternal glory that far outweighs them all. So we fix our eyes not on what is seen, but on what is unseen, since what is seen is temporary, but what is unseen is eternal.

Thank you for the continued prayers on our behalf. We love y'all. Coram DEO

9.28.2016 Update

Judy made it to a clinic visit with Dr. Erba without any side trips!!! No ambulance rides. No emergency rooms visits. No readmission to Hem/Onc floor. Just a normal visit to the clinic. I'm giddy.

As we were in the clinic hallway getting vital signs, Dr. Erba came and leaned over to Judy to whisper in her ear. He then whispered in mine that what he told Judy was a secret and he wasn't going to tell me. He went on down to the next exam room, shot one of his grins at me with a twinkle in his eye, and went in to see another patient. I looked at Judy who had tears in her eyes and she said the bone marrow biopsy, blood work, and lumbar puncture from last week showed absolutely no trace of leukemia. That currently means complete remission! Y'all…it wasn't pretty, but I did a hallway happy dance right then and there. The three nurses checking Judy's vital signs were very kind not to call the gentlemen to bring the white canvas coat with the shiny buckles and wrap around sleeves for me.

Dr. Erba went over all of last week's results with us and told Judy he was absolutely not concerned that she felt as beat down as she has been feeling and that he would expect her to feel that way due to what all she's been through in recent weeks. Due to the aggressive nature of Judy's leukemia and the goal of getting her to transplant, he and other various departmental doctors providing her care agreed that the treatment needed to be very aggressive. That's why she had the Blincyto treatment, lumbar punctures with intrathecal chemotherapy, and the Craniospinal irradiation so closely together. It was done with one goal in mind…to keep the leukemia in remission so she can get to transplant. The most recent blood workup shows no evidence of the gene mutation that was causing the leukemia to replicate so rapidly.

We also had a very frank and candid discussion with Dr. Erba where he went in to questions and answers that he felt should be asked and discussed as if he were the patient facing transplant. The most sobering discussion was one that involved the big question that Judy and I have both had since around the second month of this journey. What if all these treatments don't keep the leukemia in remission? Since it came back so rapidly in the second month, what's to keep it at bay and in remission? That's where the transplant timing became so critical and the aggressiveness of the treatment plan developed. If the cancer doesn't stay in remission, then the chances of the transplant being successful are diminished. We trust in our God and Father that His timing is perfect. He has shown us time and again over the years that at just the right time, and not a moment too soon or too late, His plan will be done. We are praying that His plan is for complete and total healing for Judy. Please join us in that prayer.

Please continue to pray for a huge turnout for the bone marrow drive in Judy's honor on October 13th at the Pelham Civic Center and Ice Arena from 3:00PM until 7:00PM. The City of Pelham is hosting this event with Be The Match Registry and we are truly humbled for their love for us. It's simply a cheek swab and fill out some paperwork. It couldn't be simpler. Our donor took the time and effort to participate in a drive in the past and we can't wait to thank him for saving Judy's life. Please participate. Thanks! Coram DEO

Chapter Seven – October 2016

10.10.2016 Update

Please pray for a huge turnout for the bone marrow drive in Judy's honor this Thursday, October 13th at the Pelham Civic Center and Ice Arena from 3:00PM until 7:00PM. The City of Pelham is hosting this event with Be The Match Registry and we are truly humbled for their love for us. It's simply a cheek swab and fill out some paperwork. It couldn't be simpler. Our donor took the time and effort to participate in a drive in the past and we can't wait to thank him for saving Judy's life. Please participate.

So what's been happening? I'm glad you asked! Last week Judy began the transplant pre-testing on Monday with a pulmonary workup, chest x-ray, and blood workup. They must have drawn about 10 to 12 vials of blood. I'm surprised she has any left! We ended up the day with a trip to the Infusion Clinic to get some IV fluids and nausea medicine. Tuesday was Matt's birthday and we loved having the kiddos and their spouses over for supper. Wednesday morning we met with Dr. Donna Salzman, the transplant doctor, to discuss the next couple of week's timeline. We also discussed starting home IV fluid therapy as this seems to help keep Judy hydrated and lower her nausea. Thursday morning Judy went to Cardiographics for an echo followed by a bone marrow biopsy that afternoon. Saturday she had a dental review and that's it until tomorrow!

Tuesday we meet with the Radiation Oncologist for mapping Judy's body for the full body radiation she'll start next week. We'll learn how Dr. Bredel wants to approach shielding the parts of her body that received

Craniospinal radiation a few weeks ago. We will meet with the transplant team Tuesday to sign all the consent papers. Judy will have some type of port placement to replace her PICC line on Friday. Saturday, Sunday & Monday she will receive pre-transplant medications and will be admitted to the Bone Marrow Transplant unit Tuesday afternoon. Full body radiation on Wednesday, Thursday, & Friday. Chemo treatments on Thursday, Friday, Saturday & Sunday. Rest day on Monday the 24th and transplant on Tuesday the 25th!!!!!!!!

So…as you can see, there are lots of opportunities for prayers over the next weeks and months of recuperation. We truly appreciate you. Coram DEO

10.15.2016 Update

When we look back over the past 6 months, we see God moving in a mighty way to bring honor and glory to His name. Placing the right doctors, nurses, nurse practitioners, technicians, insurance consultants, community, friends and family in just the right spots at just the right times to provide shoulders to cry on, spot on advice, wisdom, guidance, love, comforting words, fund raisers, prayers, etc, etc, etc. We are forever humbled by you.

The turnout for the bone marrow drive in Judy's honor this past Thursday at the Pelham Civic Center and Ice Arena hosted by the City of Pelham with Be The Match Registry was phenomenal. Twenty one new additions to the registry were added that night with others to be added through the website in the coming weeks. Thank y'all for signing up to possibly save a person's life. Well done, good and faithful servants. You can still visit Be The Match at the following site (https://join.bethematch.org/Pelham) and sign up. Just use the promo code of 'Pelham' to give credit to the City. Very special thanks to Paula Holly in the Mayor's Office for coordinating this event. She always goes above and beyond.

Tuesday morning we met with the Radiation Oncologist for mapping Judy's body for the full body radiation she'll start next week. Tuesday afternoon we met with the transplant team to sign all the consent papers. Judy had a Hickman catheter placement on Friday. Today, tomorrow & Monday she will receive pre-transplant medications and be admitted to the Bone Marrow Transplant unit late

Tuesday afternoon. Judy's full body radiation will be on Wednesday, Thursday, & Friday. Her chemo treatments will be on Friday, Saturday, Sunday and Monday. Rest day on Tuesday the 24th with bone marrow transplant on Wednesday the 26th. The dates for transplant have shifted a day due to donor needs.

So…our bags are soon to be packed and take up temporary residence at the BMT unit at UAB. Thank you for your continued prayers. Whom you have lifted your prayers to is the One that has gotten Judy into remission and brought us to the cusp of transplant. We are humbled and truly blessed. Coram DEO

10.21.2016 Update
Judy finished her radiation treatments today on day -5 and began an immunosuppressant called Atgam. The BMT staff calls it "Bunny Gam" because it is created in the thymus gland of rabbits. But due to the reaction that Judy had, instead of a cute little bunny, I think the pharmaceutical company used a Jackalope. Within about 30 minutes of infusion beginning, Judy's heart rate started spiking and her blood pressure dropped, nausea started, rigors began and her temperature rose slightly. Temp was only in the 99s however her heart rate spiked several times into the 180s & 190s with the highest topping out at 213. Her BP dropped into the 75/60 range. That's when I sent out the urgent FB request for prayer.

And y'all came through again.

As the prayers of God's people were being lifted, all vital signs started slowly returning to normal. Currently at 8:23PM, her HR is 112, BP is 110/79, nausea is gone, temp is back to normal and the rigors have stopped. You can't tell me that God doesn't hear the prayers of His warriors.

The Atgam has been suspended for the night and the doctors will reconvene in the morning to assess. We are so grateful for the BMT staff. It was a group effort and my heart is full of gratitude. They are truly God's gift for Judy's healing. Love y'all! Coram DEO

10.23.2016 Update

I need to make some corrections to the info I've put out over the last 24 to 48 hours. My FB message on Friday night asked for prayer due to Judy's reaction to the chemo. Actually it was a reaction to the Atgam that she had started and it is an immunosuppressant. Within about 30 minutes of infusion beginning Friday night, Judy's heart rate started spiking and her blood pressure dropped, nausea started, rigors began and her temperature rose slightly. Temp was only in the 99s however her heart rate spiked several times into the 180s & 190s with the highest topping out at 213. Her BP dropped into the 75/60 range. I also said that they were suspending the infusion for the night and would regroup in the morning. The doctors actually conferred that night and decided to restart the infusion, but at a much slower infusion rate. After the initial reaction, she's done very well. Evidently, everyone has a reaction to the Atgam; it's just a matter of to what degree. Today she will finish up with the Atgam & get the 3rd of 4 chemo treatments. The chemo infusions are Fludarabine and only take about 20 to 30 minutes. These she has tolerated pretty well. I'm sure glad God knew the difference in the prayer requested vs what He granted. We offer the prayers and He'll make the corrections!

We are so grateful for the BMT doctors and staff. It was a group effort and my heart is full of gratitude. They are truly God's gift for Judy's healing as are you, our friends and prayer warriors. Thank you for standing in the gap for us. Love y'all! Coram DEO

10.25.2016 Update
In my best NASA voice: We're at T -1 and ready for launch.

Last night I went to bed (well…the lovely reclining chair) thinking about Judy's donor. I prayed for him to be comforted today with a return to normalcy as rapidly as possible. I woke up this morning and he has been on my mind for most of the day. What an absolutely indescribable gift. To be willing to give the gift of life. Today, somewhere in the United States, that is exactly what this young man did for Judy. Willingly. Not even knowing her. Just willing to give a bag of marrow. Wow. Truly humbling to think what he has done.

Tomorrow on Wednesday, October 26, 2016, Judy will receive a bag of bone marrow that looks a lot like a unit of blood. Our doctor said that it'll be somewhat anticlimactic after the journey to get her to this point. It'll take about an hour to infuse and then the wait for the red & white cells as well as the platelets to start doing their thing. That timeframe will range anywhere from 10 days to a month and then we will be released home.

Over 2000 years ago, Someone Else chose to give an absolutely indescribable gift. Willingly. It was also the gift of life. Not just life on Earth. Eternal life. God chose before the beginning of the world to send His only Son. That whomever believes in Him and accepts Him into their life, would live forever. Forever. That's a really really long time. He knows our names. He stands at the door of our heart and knocks. We simply need to ask

Him in. It's a free gift that we only have to accept. Truly humbling to think what He has done.

So tomorrow is sort of a big day. Pray that all goes according to His plan. That He would continue to direct everyone involved in the transplant. That He and He alone would receive the honor and glory due His name. Coram DEO

10.31.2016 Update
T +5. And the wait continues.

Wednesday, October 26, 2016, Day 0, Judy received her donated bone marrow. The first week post transplant can and has been a somewhat up & down experience. Some days ok and others a real struggle to even get out of bed. Her blood levels have bottomed out completely. Case in point; normal White Blood Cell count for a female is between 4,000 and 11,000 units. Judy's this morning was 0.03. This means that she is very susceptible to infection hence the scrubbing and sanitizing of hands, visitor limitation, daily shower and change of clothes and bed clothing every day. She is and will continue to be on what is called a Neutropenic diet for the foreseeable future to limit the exposure to harmful bacteria and cross contamination while preparing meals.

Some of the side effects that are being watched for are changes to her mouth, pain, gastro problems, skin changes, fatigue, fluid & electrolyte imbalance, kidney problems, infection, and Graft-Versus-Host Disease. All of which will decrease as soon as her new stem cells complete what is called engraftment and the WBC, RBC & Platelets begin producing new healthy blood.

Yesterday was one of the not so good days. Extreme fatigue where all she wanted to do was sleep. And sleep she did. This woman can really snore! And she deserves to snore just as loud and proud as she wants to. Today has been a good bit better day. Woke up and wanted a shower ASAP. Sat up in the chair for a good hour.

Napped for the remainder of the morning until around midafternoon and then went for a walk in the hallway.

For all of this we are extremely thankful. Thankful that she has this disease today rather than 2 years ago. The medicine that got her into remission wasn't available 2 years ago. Thankful she didn't have this disease 10 years ago because back then she wouldn't have qualified for a transplant. Thankful that God's timing is always perfect. Always.

Please continue to pray for Judy's health and recovery. Pray that all continues according to His plan. That He would continue to direct everyone involved with the transplant and recovery. That He and He alone would receive the honor and glory due His name. Coram DEO

Chapter Eight – November 2016

11.2.2016
T +7. And it's LIMBO Day!!!!!!! How low can you go??!??

As mentioned on T +5 Judy's WBC was 0.03. This morning it's 0.01. She received a Neupogen shot yesterday to stimulate her WBC creation so we should start to see results pretty soon. So…for those of you that would like to participate in LIMBO Day…how low can you go? (this is a rhetorical question and not meant to stimulate participation from the general public)

Her oral care is probably on the top of our prayer requests at the moment. The chemo that she received both pre and post-transplant has created the mouth sores that we were told about. Judy is receiving pain meds to ease the discomfort as well as an antidote today to counteract the chemo. It's a delicate balancing act and I am fascinated with the attention that Judy, as well as all patients on the BMT Unit, receives from the doctors, NPs, nurses and PCTs. They truly are the hands and feet of Christ.

Yesterday was a pretty good day considering what all Judy has been through. Walked a couple of times. Enjoyed a smoothie that one of the nurses fixed for her. Napped a good bit. Caught up on FB and talked with family. One day at a time.

For all of this we continue to be extremely grateful & thankful. Grateful that we are one step closer to being released home. Thankful for your prayers on our behalf.

We're trying diligently to do our part. Thank you for doing yours! Coram DEO

11.9.2016 Update

T +14. The day after our nation went to the polls to cast their votes for the next leadership of this great nation. Today, half the nation is sad and half is happy. So let me offer this saying:

Hope is being able to see that there is Light, despite all the darkness. Desmond Tutu

Let's pull together as the greatest nation on earth and FIX the problems facing us. That's about as political as I'm going to get. And lest you think I'm well-read for that Tutu statement…it came off a coffee cup.

Her oral care is still on the top of our prayer requests at the moment. There's not much of a way I can describe how bad the inside of her mouth and tongue look. Imagine the brightest red of Santa Claus' coat. Not the Billy Bob Thornton 'Bad Santa' color. I mean the Coca-Cola polar bear Santa color. That's what the inside looks like; extremely painful, sore and swollen. The doctor has turned off the pain pump for about an hour and will restart at ½ the dosage Judy was getting. This is due her sleeping all the time and trying to wean her from the pain pump. She's got plenty of Magic Mouthwash to assist with pain control.

Her blood levels are starting to gradually, ever so slightly edge in the upwards direction. This morning her WBC is at 0.06. One day at a time.

Thank you for your prayers on our behalf. We're getting closer each day to going home. Coram DEO

11.12.2016 Update
T +17. Just a brief update to let you know her White
Blood Count (WBC) is headed in the right direction.

11.06.16 She was at 0.01
11.07.16 She was at 0.02
11.08.16 She was at 0.03
11.09.16 She was at 0.06
11.10.16 She was at 0.13
11.11.16 She was at 0.5
Today She is at 1.79

4 to 11 is considered normal levels.

Her oral care still needs our prayers as well as the side
effects from Tacrolimus which is the immunosuppressant
medication. She has confusion, weakness, dizziness,
lightheadedness, increased thirst, and trouble thinking
clearly. This will all clear up in the coming days. It's just
tough watching her go through it.

Thank you for your prayers on our behalf. We're getting
closer each day to going home. Coram DEO

11.15.2016 Update
T +20 and in my best Ed McMahon voice…here's your
WBC update!!!!!!!

Friday she was at 0.5
Saturday she was at 1.79
Sunday she was at 3.01
Yesterday she was at 4.7
Today, she is at **4.94** where 4 to 11 is considered normal
levels.

Her body is creating the good stuff now and we have a
target to go home of anywhere from tomorrow to the end
of this week. That's right…we'll be home for
Thanksgiving! Tomorrow was the original target date and
would have been my Dad's 91st birthday. Happy 2nd
birthday in Heaven, Pops.

The main thing holding us up is nutrition. She needs to
be able to eat and this has been difficult with the mouth
issues. These are clearing up nicely but still have a little
ways to go.

Her confusion, weakness, dizziness, lightheadedness,
increased thirst, and trouble thinking clearly are all
getting better each passing day as well.

Thank you for your prayers on our behalf. Coram DEO

11.19.2016 Update

T +24. WBC is at 15.52 which is slightly elevated and we're still waiting on her body to start accepting nutrition. The digestive tract is still recovering and we're trying to establish a routine to have nausea meds on-board prior to eating. She's able to eat a few bites of a nutritional shake that we make for her however, she starts burping a great deal. It's a balancing act that we're working on.

Even though her WBC is 15.52, the doctors are not concerned that she's harboring an infection. Judy has no fevers at any time of the day or night. Elevated levels are not uncommon with a system that is trying to reboot.

Our target to go home is still a moving goal. We've hoped to be home by Thanksgiving but we really want to be sure that Judy is setup for success and not setting her up to come right back as an in-patient. There's still the possibility, however it's a day to day decision. We'll know in plenty of time so that she's not on the street corner looking for a taxi ride home.

The care, love and attention that Judy is receiving from the staff is second to none. They are simply the best at what they do. I would love to list names of all our caregivers, but I'm sure to leave one out. So…from a very grateful heart…you know who you are and you have blessed us with your knowledge, wisdom, compassion and caring. Thank you is just not enough.

Please continue to pray for Judy's body to recover and for her strength and stamina. Coram DEO

11.20.2016 Update
T +25. The body is amazingly and delicately balanced. One little thing can domino into several things to watch. Less than an hour after I posted yesterday, her temperature spiked into the 100s, her kidneys are 'unhappy' (doctor's words), and her urine output is close to zero. She has the urge to go however, very little if anything happens.

So…she's started back on antibiotics, had 2 chest x-rays, drawn blood cultures, and an ultrasound of her bladder. And on top of all this…she fell trying to use the bedside toilet. While she was sleeping, I had gone to the family restroom to shower and when I returned, I found her on the floor. Nothing serious, just her legs gave way from being so weak and she buckled to the floor. Thankfully she did not hit her head or we would be looking at a whole different ballgame. So for now, we're utilizing the bedpan and the bed alarm is set.

We're not sure what this does to our target to go home. I'd sure rather enjoy my turkey & dressing rather than the institutional version! But the timeline to get home is still and always has been in God's Hands. His timing is always perfect. Never delayed. Never incorrect. Never altered. Always perfect.

Thank you for your continued prayers. Please continue to pray for Judy's body to recover and for her strength and stamina. And while you're at it, please thank God for His prefect timing. Coram DEO

11.24.2016 Update

I'm thankful for this new day. I'm thankful that Judy is such a fighter. I'm thankful for God's grace, abundantly given but never deserved. I'm thankful for His wisdom that He grants to Judy's caregivers. I'm thankful for their compassionate care. I'm thankful for their observation skills where they notice more in a glance than most people do while staring. I'm thankful for our Hunter Street family that loves us and checks on us daily. I'm thankful I'm not a Butterball turkey (although I'm shaped like one). I'm thankful for family and friends that are concerned we'll have to eat institutional turkey instead of home cooked. I'm thankful for our doctors and the years of study they've put in. I'm thankful for early morning, mid-morning & late morning naps. I'm thankful for afternoon ones too. I'm thankful for handholding in the middle of the night. I'm thankful for God's guidance through this journey. I'm thankful for the peace that passes all understanding. I'm thankful for y'all reading my ramblings and praying for Judy's healing. I'm thankful for trying to live…Coram DEO.

Chapter Nine – December 2016

12.1.2016 Update
Welcome to the "December To Remember Big Event"!!!
Please note that no Lexus was harmed in the making of
this update. And we're not giving one away for free.

T+36. Wow. It's been 11 days since an update on Judy
and as she has done in exemplary fashion to date, she's
trying to let all of the medical disciplines at UAB have a
shot at practicing medicine with her. Hematology,
Oncology, Physical Therapy, Occupational Therapy,
Radiology, Pharmacy, Otolaryngology, Nephrology,
Nursing, Ophthalmology, Nutrition, Infectious Disease,
& Audiology. She's always been an overachiever.

So…Her kidneys are now happy again and output is back
in the normal range. No pain for several days other than
mild headache. Throat and mouth are clearing up nicely.
Appetite still sucks. Exercise is improving. She is
showing some high range hearing loss probably due to
radiation that we hope will clear up over time. She's had
a muscle in her right neck swell and it has the doctors
stumped as to why (again, she's allowing the doctors to
utilize all of their medical training). Physical Therapy has
her walking to the end of the unit hallway and back twice
daily, so leg strength is getting better. Fluid has built up
behind her right lung that they're watching.

As mentioned above, her appetite is really poor. She
currently is on calorie count to see if she is taking in
enough nutrition to sustain her. If not, then we're looking
at the possibility of TPN feeding or even a feeding tube
directly into the gut. We really don't want to go this route
as it will open up a whole host of possibilities for issues

we'd rather not have to deal with. Please offer prayers for this issue.

We had a stair lift installed at home in order to aid in getting Judy from the main level to the bedrooms. We've discussed one for a couple of years thinking I'd be the one to need it for my knees or hip. So in the future, if I ever do need one, Judy has been nice enough to say I can use hers. In addition to the stair lift, we have a wonderful ministry at Hunter Street called Helping Hands that will be building a wheelchair ramp this weekend for Judy. I've had the pleasure of watching these guys and their craftsmanship over the years and we are truly blessed to be on the receiving end of their skills. We are grateful for their knowledge and servants hearts.

Please continue to pray for Judy's body to recover and for her strength, stamina and appetite. Pray for protection and good weather for the Helping Hands guys. Pray that all the departments at UAB are gaining wisdom from Judy's care in order to assist others in the future. Coram DEO

12.8.2016 Update
Before today's update, I need to convey some potentially devastating news. The annual McCoy Christmas card and update letter will **not** be sent out this year. I know. I know. I've got tears as well.

T+43. In addition to the medical disciplines of Hematology, Oncology, Physical Therapy, Occupational Therapy, Radiology, Pharmacy, Otolaryngology, Nephrology, Nursing, Ophthalmology, Nutrition, Infectious Disease, & Audiology that have already had a crack at Judy, we can now add Speech Therapy. She had a swallow test this afternoon to assess how she is processing different type of solids and liquids. The Speech Therapist made some recommendations to the doctor this afternoon and she has had a feeding tube placed. Judy is totally fine with this as she knows this is the proper direction to take in order for her continued healing to take place.

Exercise and movement is improving daily. Physical Therapy has her walking to the end of the unit hallway and back twice daily, so leg strength is getting better. The fluid that was behind her right lung was drained this past Saturday. 1.5 liters were pulled off. It has been sent to culture that can take anywhere from 2 to 3 months to get a result. This is to try and determine the source of the right side neck swelling. It's like the old Johnny Carson Show where they used to play Stump the Band with Doc, Ed & Johnny. The doctors are really stumped at this time so the testing continues!

If you follow along on Facebook you may have seen pictures that Judy was granted a hall pass yesterday afternoon. This is the first time that she has been off the BMT unit since admission on October 18. Judy and I along with our son and her brother were able to go over to the atrium for 2 1/2 hours to laugh and enjoy actually looking out a window that has a view. Coupled along with the hall pass is the absolutely awesome news that:

WE MAY GET RELEASED HOME ON MONDAY THE 12TH!!!!!!!

Plans are being made and Monday is the current target date to move from in-patient to out-patient status. It has been an incredibly long and difficult journey to get Judy to this stage of recovery. Since last weekend, she has really been expressing the desire to get home. We have the necessary tools in place to aid in the successful transition home from being at UAB for so long. We thank you for the prayers that have been daily lifted for Judy and the rest of our family. To God be the glory. Great things He has done (and continues to do). Coram DEO

12.18.2016 Update

T+53. I'd like to apologize for the delay in a recent update, but it's been a bit hectic. So here goes…

WE GOT RELEASED HOME ON MONDAY THE 12TH!!!!!!!

The day after our last update 10 days ago, Judy had a Dobhoff feeding tube placed. Currently she is receiving nourishment 24 hours a day. She is also receiving her medications through this tube as well. I've spent the last week trying to hit my stride in the timing of all her medications, IV infusions of 2 medications, bathing, tooth brushing, clinic visits, restroom breaks, naps and overnight visits to the BMT Unit.

We had our first outpatient visit on Wednesday that ended up as an overnight stay. This was due to a couple of things. One was the fluid around her right lung had come back and pulmonary was booked solid Wednesday afternoon. The second was so an oxygen study to prove that Judy needed oxygen in the home setting could be completed. So…the overnight 24 hour observation showed that she does have the need and that was set up for home use. Pulmonary was there Thursday morning at 8:15am and pulled off an additional 950ml from the right lung. She has been resting much more comfortably since being released back home on Thursday.

Our next clinic visit was yesterday (Saturday) and we were there only long enough to get labs drawn and then headed right back home. But since we're basically very needy people and missed all our newest friends on the BMT floor, we decided we needed some additional excitement in our lives. This excitement manifested itself by pulling Judy's feeding tube all the way out! Yeah us! On the way to one of our restroom breaks, the feeding tube line got tangled in the wheels of the walker and you can guess the rest. So…we loaded back up and headed back to UAB to have a new feeding tube placed. The newest tube is now safety-pinned in two locations on her pajamas so if it comes out this time…clothes are coming off with it.

Judy's lab values have been looking very good. We are thankful that recovery, despite the side trips, is going very well. I'm thankful for the training that was shown to me prior to Judy's release. Thankful for a beautiful wheelchair ramp to get her up to the house. Thankful for a stair lift to get her to her bedroom. Thankful for your continued prayers. Thankful that we can and will celebrate 37 years of marriage this coming Thursday. Thankful for this time of year that we celebrate the birth of our Lord and Saviour. Coram DEO

12.28.2016 Update
T+63. How about a post-Christmas/pre-New Year update?

Judy passed her swallow retest on Thursday the 22nd and the feeding tube was officially removed on purpose (not by our clumsiness) by the BMT outpatient staff that day which was our 37th wedding anniversary. We had a very quiet anniversary and Christmas at home. We slept through several Hallmark Christmas movies and really enjoyed being home. Jennifer and Phillip came over Sunday night for supper. We'll have our big Christmas dinner this weekend when Matt and Charlie return from Atlanta (pending Judy being home).

Yesterday was Tuesday the 28th and we had a regular outpatient clinic visit scheduled. The 2 prior nights at home, Judy had been having increasing difficulty with shortness of breath after mild exertion. We had a CT done on her lungs which showed that fluid was building up again, particularly around her right lung. Due this, we were readmitted yesterday afternoon with the plan to consult in Pulmonary to run more extensive testing to determine the cause and source of the fluid recurrence. One of the Pulmonary doctors just left and the plan is to have another thoracentesis done this afternoon. The results will be sent for extensive testing and comparison to the previous tests. Also sometime this week, Judy will have a procedure done to examine the interior of her lung and biopsy a portion of the inflammation. Please pray this procedure will clearly reveal what has been going on with her lungs and the fluid buildup throughout her body.

Also she will have an echo test on the heart since the CT showed some fluid there as well.

Judy's lab values continue to look very good. As we approach the New Year, we are confident in this one thing: That He Who began a good work in us, will see it through to completion until the day of Christ Jesus. To Him be all honor, glory and praise. Coram DEO

Chapter Ten – January 2017

1.6.2017 Update

T+72. Happy New Year!

We're still in-patient at the moment. The fluid removed from the thoracentesis Wednesday the 28th still is not showing any indications of infection. As such, a more aggressive approach will now be taken. Thoracic Surgery is now being consulted to possibly perform a thoracoscopic surgery. During this procedure, a chest tube will be inserted to drain the accumulated fluid in Judy's lung and a portion of her lung will be removed and sent for biopsy. This will hopefully reveal the source of the fluid buildup. Please pray that it will definitively reveal what is going on. So…not to worry…we're not out running the roads during Winter Storm 2017 or looking for places to slide down hills. We'll be here at UAB for the next little bit.

Judy continues to improve both in strength as well as appetite each day. We still have a long way to go with eating, but she didn't arrive at this point overnight either. It'll be a while before she's back to full appetite.

Judy's lab values continue to improve and head in the right direction. As we enter the New Year, we are confident in this one thing: That He Who began a good work in us, will see it through to completion until the day of Christ Jesus. To Him be all honor, glory and praise. Thank you for your continued prayers on Judy's behalf. Coram DEO

01.13.2017 Update

In my very best German accent…V.A.T.S. that you say?

We're still in-patient! This past Monday, Judy had a VATS which is a video-assisted thoracoscopic surgery. A small incision was made in the right side of her chest and surgical instruments inserted. The surgeon removed 2 liters of fluid, biopsied some of the lung, sprayed talc & antibiotics onto the plural wall to aid with lung adhesion, and inserted the chest drain tube. So far, the preliminary reports are all negative. Reports can take from 3 days to a month or more depending on the complexity of the test. The current thinking is that Judy may have a mild case of GVHD…Graft vs Host Disease. This is when the donated cells can begin to attack the recipient's normal cells. It can range from mild to moderate to severe to even life threatening. Please understand that even if it is determined to be GVHD, that it is a very mild case that can be successfully treated with antibiotics, steroids, and inhalers. We hope to know more in the coming days.

Judy had her catheter removed today and we're hoping the chest tube will be removed tomorrow. The drainage needs to reduce to a certain level before the surgical team is comfortable with removal. We were close this morning so we're hopeful that tomorrow Judy will be tube free. Currently we are moving towards release home at the beginning of the week.

Nutritional needs are back on the discussion table as well. She is being given a couple of different appetite stimulants. So far, the further she gets away from Monday's surgery and reduction in the need for pain medicine, the better she is eating. Tonight for supper she ate all of her chicken salad and 95% of her fruit cup.

Please pray for the above mentioned items. We truly appreciate, need, and covet them. Thank you for interceding on Judy's behalf. Coram DEO

Chapter Eleven – February 2017

02.01.2017 Update

Welcome to February which is Judy's birth month. Let the celebration begin!

It was back on day + 79 when last we updated. Today is day +98. So…let's get everyone caught up.

We've been home for over a week now which has to be some kind of record for Judy to stay out-patient! Seems like we've just gotten home in the past just in time to turn around and head back in. It's been wonderful to sleep in our own bed. We were released on day +89 and we're shooting for over a month before a particular treatment begins that will require Judy to be in-patient for a few days. We go to out-patient clinic twice a week for blood workups and occasional IV infusions.

The VATS (video-assisted thoracoscopic surgery) was very successful. The chest tube was removed on day +84 and the lung fluid has not resurfaced. The current thinking is that she had a mild case of GVHD…Graft vs Host Disease. This is when the donated cells can begin to attack the recipient's normal cells. It can range from mild to moderate to severe to even life threatening. We've started treatment with antibiotics & steroids. Judy hasn't hit me over the head with a chair so I'm confident that 'Roid Rage hasn't set in yet.

The current plan is to remain out-patient for at least a month before we start a maintenance dose of Blincyto. This is the medication (along with much prayer) that got Judy into remission. We'll have a Bone Marrow Biopsy tomorrow with Lumbar Punctures set to begin in about another month. These are the 2 main tests that determine that the leukemia is still in remission. Currently, one of the blood tests shows that Judy's blood is 100% donor, which is excellent.

Matt and Charlie have been house and dog sitting for us for several months. They will be moving to an apartment in Homewood in the next couple of weeks. I don't think they truly understand how much they have helped us since last April. Also Lisa and Harold Emmons have stepped in at the drop of a telephone call. They all have truly been the hands and feet of Christ. Judy and I will be forever grateful.

Thank you for the phone calls, texts, visits, gift cards, and especially prayers. We appreciate every single one of them. Coram DEO

02.06.2017 Update

Well folks, there's no other way to convey this information. The Bone Marrow Biopsy last Thursday shows that Judy's cancer has returned. The leukemia has a different genetic marker that will not allow the use of the Blincyto. The Blincyto targeted the CD19 genetic marker and the latest tests show that marker CD22 is the new target.

We are exploring options to include possible clinical trials in either Nashville at Sarah Cannon Research Institute or Houston at MD Anderson. Judy would have to qualify for these studies. The other option is hospice.

Please pray that we would have clarity in our decision making. We appreciate every single one of your prayers. Coram DEO

02.13.2017 Update

Today was our regular doctor outpatient visit. We were able to discuss in detail the options that are available to explore for Judy's continued treatment. Here's what we know at the moment:

There are not any treatment options available at UAB. The Jakafi medication is a possibility, however Dr. Erba and Dr. Salzman feel like a better chance for long term viability is with the investigational medicine treatments at MD Anderson. Dr. Erba has provided a contact in Houston that we are attempting to follow up with. I've submitted an online referral request to MD Anderson and I expect to hear from them tomorrow (Tuesday). Dr. Salzman has also sent an email, so, we'll see if there are any research trials available and if Judy qualifies for one.

Our friends in Houston have been absolutely phenomenal to us. Offers to stay at their homes, offers of contacts for long term apartments, flat out offers of being at our service for whatever we need. This is so very comforting to us to be surrounded by such a great crowd of witnesses to help us run this race. We will persevere.

Our current fervent prayer is that Judy will qualify for a research trial. Please pray for a rapid referral. Please pray that we would have clarity in our decision making. We appreciate every single one of your prayers. Coram DEO

02.15.2017 Update

Ephesians 5:19-20 says:

> ***Speaking to one another with psalms, hymns, and songs from the Spirit. Sing and make music from your heart to the Lord, always giving thanks to God the Father for everything, in the name of our Lord Jesus Christ.***

We give thanks to God our Father as we are confirmed to see Dr. Farhad Ravandi at MD Anderson on Monday, February 27th at 1:30PM! Our first appointment that day is with Registration at 9:00AM. Judy will have a test at 9:30AM and meet with Dr. Ravandi at 1:30PM. MD Anderson has asked us to plan to be in Houston for at least 3 to 5 days post appointment in the event additional testing is needed.

We are having Judy's medical records, chemistry panels, Bone Marrow Biopsy pathology, and blood tests sent to them for review. We are also considering our options for travel to Houston. We have an extremely generous offer to fly us there. We are also looking at driving over a couple of days because of the mobility equipment Judy needs to navigate (i.e. Rollator, walker, wheelchair, etc.) Throw in sleeping arrangements and we have a plethora of decisions to make. (I wanted to say plethora, so roll with me here.)

With all of the walls that God has crumbled for us to get this appointment, we are confident that He knows the plans He has for us. I just hope I'm listening close enough to what we need to do and be the safest form of travel for Judy.

Please be in prayer tomorrow evening (Thursday) around 5:30PM as we will be having a prayer service for Judy. The 5th chapter of James verses 13 through 16 says that we are to call on the elders of the church to pray and anoint with oil and the prayer of faith will save the sick. That is our fervent prayer. Please lift her up at this time. Coram DEO

02.21.2017 Update

Our bags are getting packed and we're ready to head to Houston! We have decided to drive as we feel that will be the safest and most comfortable for Judy. My favorite sister, Marcy (read…my only sister), is flying in to Birmingham Thursday to help drive. We're leaving on Friday to Baton Rouge, which is about halfway and continue on in to Houston on Saturday. That will give us Sunday to rest and prepare for Monday. We have wonderful friends that have offered for us to stay with them. As soon as we wear out our welcome with them, we've had other offers to stay with as well. So…if you don't see Judy's Big Black Truck pulling into your driveway Saturday, rest easy, you still may get a chance to host the traveling circus.

Our first appointment Monday is with Registration at 9:00AM. Judy will begin testing at 9:30AM and meet with Dr. Ravandi at 1:30PM. MD Anderson has asked us to plan to be in Houston for at least 3 to 5 days post appointment in the event additional testing is needed. They have received all necessary medical records and we've filled out a good portion of demographic info online which I'm hoping will speed the registration process.

With all of the walls that God has crumbled for us to get this appointment, we are confident that He knows the plans He has for us. There are still a bunch (I'm giving plethora a rest this update) of unanswered questions at this point. How long will we be in Houston? Will Judy qualify for a clinical trial? Will treatment start immediately or will we head back to Birmingham first?

What are the side effects of the treatment should Judy qualify? But because God holds us in the palm of His hand, these and other questions I haven't thought of yet are already answered. They will be revealed to us at exactly the appropriate time and not a moment too soon.

Please be in prayer for safe travels and Judy's fatigue level. Offer prayers of thanksgiving and gratitude for Bill & Donna Dagley for graciously opening their home to us. Pray for Judy's new Houston medical team. Offer additional prayers of thanksgiving for our phenomenal care team at UAB. Offer praise to Him Who is able. Coram DEO

02.27.2017 Update

Our travel to Houston went extremely well. Judy was an absolute trooper. We left Friday and drove to Baton Rouge for the night and on in to Houston on Saturday. We rested well yesterday and hit the ground running this morning.

Our first appointment was with Registration at 9:00AM. Judy had blood workups (17 vials) at 9:30AM and met with Dr. Ravandi at 1:00PM. We met with a clinical research nurse to discuss a possible trial that Judy can participate in if her blood work & bone marrow biopsy match her records from UAB. After that meeting, we had the bone marrow biopsy and a chest x-ray. Whew!

So…with all that said, we do have hope in the fact that options are available which also include treatment without the clinical trial. We go back Wednesday & Friday of this week for more blood work. We hope to have the bone marrow biopsy results as early as Friday, but may be next Monday. We meet with Dr. Ravandi again on Monday.

Thank you for your prayers on Judy's behalf. They are being heard and acted upon. Please continue to offer praise to Him Who is able. Coram DEO

02.29.2017 Update

Brief update on Judy. Early this AM she awoke with a high fever and mental confusion. She was admitted late this afternoon to MD Anderson after arriving this morning through the ER. She has received large doses of fluids all day coupled with electrolytes. Additional blood work as well as CT & chest x-ray have been completed. We haven't heard results yet.

In addition to all this, our hosts Bill & Donna Dagley are also in the hospital with Bill having health complications as well. Please pray for Bill & Judy's medical teams for clarity, understanding, insight, compassion, and whatever else you'd like to add. Also...please please please pray for our housing situation. Donna has the gift of hospitality and still offers her home in addition to caring for Bill. Judy & I have decided to look closer in around the Texas Medical Center for either a hotel room or short term stay apartment. We truly appreciate the Dagley's and felt like we couldn't continue to take advantage of their hospitality when Bill is dealing with his issues as well.

So much for a brief update but, that's the latest. We'll update as more becomes available. Coram DEO

UPDATE...Most of the housing issue this week is rodeo is in town. We're already on several waiting lists for first come first served.

Chapter Twelve – March 2017

03.01.2017 Update

After Judy was admitted late yesterday to MD Anderson, she rested comfortably in between all the hourly checks. The fever has abated and the mental confusion is better as well. Today, she has been ordering her own food from room service, has already had Physical Therapy and Occupational Therapy is currently here for assessment. When I got here this morning, I missed the doctor by about 10 minutes. However, it appears that Judy has a treatment plan that may start as soon as tomorrow! She has been approved for a clinical trial and we are absolutely thrilled that there are options available.

When I asked yesterday for y'all to please (please please) pray for our housing situation, WOW did God open the floodgates. Many of the websites that y'all sent I had already been given by the case manager. Since the rodeo is in town, the case manager was a bit peeved that most of the rooms that are supposed to be blocked for medical patients were snatched up by cowboys and cowgirls. But God had different plans for us. Through contacts from good ole Greenville, Mississippi friends, I'm going to look at not just one but two different locations tomorrow morning. One is a guest house about 2 miles from the medical center and the other is an apartment over around the Galleria. When God answers our prayers, He absolutely showers us with goodness and grace. Thank you Lord.

Thank you for your prayers. He listens and He answers. Every. Single. Time. Coram DEO

03.02.2017 Update

The Doxology was a short hymn of praise that we learned way back at First Presbyterian Church of Greenville, Mississippi. (or to those of us reared there…Grenvul Misipi)

Praise God, from whom all blessings flow;
Praise Him, all creatures here below;
Praise Him above, ye heavenly host;
Praise Father, Son, and Holy Ghost. Amen.

And for our musical friends, you had to hold the Amen (pronounced Ah-Men) for a 12 count or until you ran out of breath. The reason I mention this is because of the intertwining of Catechism students from that little church, way back when. There was a young lady my age, whose family were friends of mine growing up in the 1960s and 70s. Fast forward to today. This lady referred us to friends of hers whom she attends church with here in Houston. I met with the gentleman this morning to take a look at the guest house that is 2 miles from MD Anderson. And it's perfect. And we get to stay there as long as we need. FOR FREE. When I asked him why they would offer something like this at no charge, he responded that it was their way of showing God's grace that had been shown to them. Amen and amen.

Judy will begin the clinical trial this afternoon which involves a combination therapy of Jakafi and Hyper-CVAD chemo. Please pray for her strength and tolerance of the medication. The current plan is to remain in-patient for about a week and transition to out-patient for about three weeks. Another bone marrow biopsy will be performed at that time to determine if she is back in remission.

Thank you LORD for showering us with goodness and grace. Both of which are totally undeserved. Thank you for your continued intercessory prayers. He listens and He answers. Every. Single. Time. Coram DEO

03.06.2017 Update
Good Morning from Planet Houston! (For the uninitiated, that's a reference to a Superman movie)

As mentioned in a FB post from this past Saturday, Judy was released from MD Anderson to out-patient status. We spent Sunday as a day of rest, lying around this cute guest house, relaxing, napping and then late afternoon, Judy wanted ice cream. So we went to supper at Luby's Cafeteria and then to Marble Slab Creamery for ice cream. As you have probably heard…everything is bigger in Texas. Well…you should have seen the rain storm going on with us getting Judy, Rollator, purse, me, and umbrella from the guest house to the truck. I'm hoping none of the neighbors was YouTubing it.

Judy is well tolerating the Jakafi (or Ruxolitinib for those of you can pronounce it) treatment. She takes 4 pills morning and night as well as a BUNCH of other medications. She has NOT started the Hyper-CVAD treatment. I think if I'm reading the trial paperwork correctly, that if the Jakafi works, then she will not have to go through that nasty stuff. We go for blood work at 1:00 this afternoon and see Dr. Ravandi at 3:00. I think this will be our normal pattern on Monday, Wednesday & Fridays for out-patient clinic visits.

Thank you again for your continued intercessory prayers. He listens and He answers. Every. Single. Time. Coram DEO

03.16.2017 Update
Good Morning from Houston, home of the Houston Livestock Show and Rodeo since 1931!! You know it's a big deal when your hospital messaging system sends out reminders about traffic during the event.

Raise your hand if you LOVE waiting. Anyone? Bueller? Bueller? That's how Judy feels each Monday, Wednesday, and Friday goes. Our usual pattern is wait to be called to lab for blood work, wait to be called for vital signs to be taken, wait even longer for the test results to come back, and wait for test results review with either a PA or NP. We hold our breath at that point to see if we have to wait further for any fluids or platelets to be infused. Wash, rinse, repeat. But I do have to say that overall, Judy is doing extremely well with the Jakafi treatment. We should finish up the round of pills next Wednesday. She is scheduled for a bone marrow biopsy that day as well as review with Dr. Ravandi and the research team. Lots of decisions to make after the results of the bone marrow biopsy come back.

But I'd like to say something about the wait time that I've observed. In this waiting room full of strangers thrown together by damnable diseases, there are certain looks that caregivers give other caregivers. There are certain looks that cancer fighters give other cancer fighters. It's a forged bond among complete strangers that says…I know what you're dealing with, I know the fears you're facing, I know the struggles you're trying to balance, and a hundred other glances that are completely understood by people on the same path. So…how do I approach the wait times? Talk & laugh. Reach out with a smile and a nod. Use words if they seem appropriate. Get to know others from different areas of the world. Houston has always been a multi-cultural city and the waiting room is a great snapshot that reflects that.

So…we wait and we nod and we laugh and we tear up with other kindred folk walking similar but different paths. We try to spread the love of Christ, sometimes with words, sometimes without. And we pray that the message that we have eternal hope gets across. Coram DEO

03.22.2017 Update

Howdy up to ya there FB neighbors! We're heading in to the home stretch of the Houston Livestock Show & Rodeo for 2017. Guess I'll have to hang up my dingle-bob spurs till next year because we didn't get to attend any events.

Judy had a bone marrow aspiration on Monday and we met with Dr. Ravandi and the research team today. The Jakafi appears to be working in the proper direction. When we arrived at MD Anderson on February 27th, the first bone marrow showed 47% blasts circulating. That number is down to 17% after 21 days of Jakafi only treatment. Judy started the Hyper-CVAD chemo treatment tonight in combination with the Jakafi. She'll be in-patient for about 5 days and then released to out-patient status again.

So…about another month of treatment to see if we can get Judy into remission. Adult onset ALL is extremely rare and very difficult to achieve and stay in remission. But this Hyper-CVAD is a step that Judy feels like she has to take in order to complete what she set out to accomplish. Several additional vials of blood have been drawn for future research in the hopes that the next person will have an easier path to follow.

So…please pray for Judy's favorable toleration of the chemo. Coram DEO

03.29.2017 Update

Mid-week greetings from Planet Houston!

Judy transitioned back to out-patient status yesterday after beginning her in-patient chemo treatment. She will have a couple of well-deserved rest days before going to clinic on Friday. We got to the guest house around 5:30 yesterday afternoon and she's been asleep practically ever since. So…I'm drinking coffee and watching the sawdust gather around her bed from all the log sawing going on.

We'll go in Saturday around noon for another portion of the Hyper-CVAD treatment. This one is the 'V' portion and can be given on an out-patient basis. She will also start the 'D' portion on Saturday as well but this is 5 tablets that she takes at home for 4 days. Overall she is tolerating the treatments very well. Mild nausea so far but seems to have settled down enough for her to get some well-deserved rest.

The preliminary reports from her Lumbar Punctures show that there is no CNS involvement of the leukemia. This means it hasn't made the jump across the blood/brain barrier to involve the spinal fluid and brain. Praise the Lord. She did have CNS involvement back in Birmingham which brought about the radiation treatments. We are very thankful for this as she doesn't want to undergo those kinds of treatments ever again. Let me rephrase that…she has stated she will NOT do that again. Most of the long term side effects she's dealing with can be traced to the radiation. Nasty nasty stuff.

So…we'll be here in Houston until the doctor visit on April 12th. We will be released home to Pelham and continued follow-up with Dr. Erba at The Kirklan Clinic and/or Dr. Salzman at BMT at that point. Oh to feel the sheets on our own bed!

I need to give a very special shout out to the Mellow Mushroom restaurant & the Good People Brewing Company for their spectacular fundraising efforts on Judy's behalf. WOW what a success. To date it's the largest fundraising effort for MM. If you're in the area, please continue to grace them with your dining dollars. They are more than deserving.

So…please pray for Judy's continued favorable toleration of the chemo. Please pray also for our release and homecoming in April. Coram DEO

Chapter Thirteen – April 2017

4.1.2017 Update

The reason for my #CancerSucks Facebook post yesterday is due to Judy being readmitted to in-patient status. We went in for a regular clinic visit Friday and her blood pressure was so low that they took her immediately to the Emergency Room. Chest x-ray, stomach CT, blood cultures, flu swab, bags of fluid, bags of antibiotics, etc, etc, etc. She was admitted last night and the consensus is that everything is pointing at severe dehydration due to chemo induced diarrhea. The Hyper-CVAD treatment coupled with the trial medication seems to be the culprit. After being released this past Tuesday, I gave her a bag of IV fluid on Wednesday here at the guest house in addition to the 3 bottles of water she consumed. Thursday, it was 4 bottles consumed. The doctors said there really wasn't anything we could have done differently at home. So...she's back in-patient for the next few days which is really ok with both of us. She had the Vincristine treatment today as well as starting the Dexamethasone. If this contributes to additional episodes of diarrhea, then she is exactly in the correct place. Please pray for her strength and endurance. This is a very tough race to run. Much love to y'all. Coram DEO

04.07.2017 Update
Happy Friday Everyone! Things are happening so quickly that it's hard to keep up and keep everyone informed. But here goes:

After only two days at the guest house, we went in to what we thought would be a normal clinic visit last Friday. Judy's blood pressure was extremely low and the clinic staff immediately took her to the emergency room. She was extremely dehydrated. After the 3rd & 4th portions of the Hyper-CVAD treatment over the weekend, the beginning of this week brought the news of the sepsis. She was initially responding to the antibiotics however, a 3rd bacterium has presented and she has digressed considerably. The past couple of days have been the hardest for me to watch. Judy is having trouble communicating now. Her words are getting stuck and won't come out. A CT was performed two days ago to rule out a brain bleed. Neurology was consulted in yesterday, an EEG performed, and results sent for review. An MRI will probably be performed today.

We are scheduled to see Dr. Ravandi next Wednesday as that is the 21st day of this treatment cycle. But that appointment is questionable due to Judy's in-patient status. We were hoping to be released back to Birmingham at that time, however, we'll just have to wait and see how the infection control goes. I'm beginning the research into corporate Angel flights back to Birmingham. Judy is in such a weakened state that I think it would be vastly easier on her rather than 2 days travelling by vehicle. I know one of our former student ministry kids works for a Med-Jet type practice and if you know their name…toss me a bone because I can't remember who!

So…lots of requests to ask you to bring before the throne of grace. Mercy. Intervention. Guidance. Grace. Peace. Tranquility. Healing. Calmness…You get the picture. Thank you for your loving support of us. Your love and prayers are sustaining us. Coram DEO

04.09.2017 Update

Happy Palm Sunday everyone, the beginning of Holy Week for Christians the world over. Our hope is built on nothing less than Jesus' blood and righteousness.

We have some less than positive news to convey this Sunday morning. The results of Judy's MRI show leukemic activity in the frontal lobe of her brain. An EEG of the brain that was performed indicated continuous non-convulsive seizures that are now being regulated with anti-seizure medication. She is not under any sedation but is non-responsive to verbal commands. She is not in any pain. There will be a lumbar puncture performed tomorrow with intrathecal chemo to see if the brain responds. This will help confirm the leukemic activity. Whether the leukemia is or isn't in her brain, her chances for recovery short of God's intervention and miracle, are not good.

Judy made the decision years ago to donate her body to medical science as she had the opportunity to train with medical cadavers at Physical Therapy school. She was accepted to UAB's Anatomical Donation program; however, death out-of-state negates the donation. The good news is that University of Texas Health Sciences Services will honor Judy's wishes and accept her body for research and training.

Y'all were so very helpful with information on Critical Care transport back to Birmingham from Houston. The former student that I couldn't remember was our very own Josh Decker, son of some guy in the front office at Hunter Street. Josh was incredibly helpful with info and guidance. I wish the situation was such that we could use this option.

Tomorrow will bring lots of things together. The full team following Judy will be back together from the weekend and we should have all the weekend testing results by then. Difficult decisions will need to be made at that point and I solicit your prayers for guidance. Judy does have Advanced Directives on file with the hospital and we will honor those directives.

So again…lots of requests to ask you to bring before the throne of grace. Mercy. Intervention. Guidance. Grace. Peace. Tranquility. Healing. Calmness…You get the picture. Thank you for your loving support of us. Your love and prayers are sustaining us. Coram DEO

4.10.2017
And now...she's responding to her name, moving her head
yes & no to questions, squeezing hands on command.
But still barely opening her eyes. Praise our good
good God.

Lumbar puncture today. Bone marrow biopsy tomorrow.
Decisions delayed until probably tomorrow as well.
Prognosis still on the not so good side.
Thanks for the prayers! Coram DEO

04.12.2017 Update

Holy, Holy, Holy, Lord God Almighty. Early in the morning, our song will rise to Thee.

The information from the Leukemia and ICU teams this morning was not good. The Bone Marrow Biopsy shows that there are 56% blasts in Judy's blood. This means that there is nothing else that can be done for her. The doctors indicated that less than 1% of people with Judy's type of leukemia and her current condition ever make it out of the hospital.

As such, the family is flying in tomorrow and comfort measures will be instituted.

Thank you for your constant prayers that have carried us through this journey. Please pray that Judy's entrance into eternity will be peaceful and quick.

2 Timothy 4: 6-8:

For I am already being poured out like a drink offering, and the time for my departure is near. I have fought the good fight, I have finished the race, I have kept the faith. Now there is in store for me the crown of righteousness, which the Lord, the righteous Judge, will award to me on that day—and not only to me, but also to all who have longed for his appearing.

Coram DEO

04.14.2017 Update

On Good Friday 2017, April 14 @ 4:54 A.M., surrounded by her family, Judy McCoy left this earth and entered eternity. Praise God from Whom all blessings flow. Well done, good and faithful servant. Enter into your reward. Coram DEO

04.26.2017 Update

A life well lived celebration will be held on Saturday, May 6, 2017 at Hunter Street Baptist Church in Hoover, AL in the Worship Center. Visitation with the family will be held from 9:30 to 11:00am with Celebration Service at 11:00. Additional visitation with the family will be available after the service. Coram DEO

Chapter Fourteen – May 2017

05.08.2017 Update

A life well lived celebration was held on Saturday, May 6, 2017 at Hunter Street Baptist Church in Hoover, AL in the Worship Center for Judy McCoy. To look out over the gathered crowd of friends and family, it was evident to me and our family just what an impact one person committed to Jesus Christ can and did have. Judy lived life to the fullest and faced each new day with an enthusiasm that can only come from an intimate knowledge of what she was placed here on this earth to do. She wanted everyone she met to have this same joy of living that she exhibited. Did she have trials and issues that she dealt with? Absolutely! Cancer can and does devastate a body. It took a vibrant healthy woman and turned her body into what appeared to be a shell of her former self. But her outward appearance wasn't Judy. Judy possessed a spirit that continues to live on in our memories and in the precious lives of our two children Matt and Jennifer as well as their spouses, Charlie and Phillip. Judy had a great joy in knowing that they all know and love the same Lord that she did for so many years.

I'm sure that there were several that wondered where the casket was at the memorial service. The answer is that there wasn't one. Judy, as she had done throughout her career as a Physical Therapist, gave of herself in death by donating her body to science. She had the opportunity to study a medical cadaver while in PT school and she wanted to give back like someone before her had done. She also knew that she would have a new body that was perfect in a way that we can only imagine. No disease. No decay. No imperfections. No aging. Healed and wholly perfect.

I wanted to thank each and every one of you that prayed for us during this past year of medical treatment. Your prayers, cards, texts, telephone calls, lawn mowed, dogs cared for, ramp built, gift cards, meals delivered, etc, etc, etc, sustained us during Judy's Journey. And please know that your prayers were completely and totally heard and completely and totally answered on April 14, 2017 at 4:54am when God spoke one word:

Healed

Coram DEO

Chapter Fifteen – March 2018

03.14.2018 Update
Happy Pi Day everyone! I wrote portions of the following update one year ago not knowing at the time that Judy only had 30 days remaining on this earth.

Raise your hand if you LOVE waiting. Anyone? Bueller? Bueller? That's how Judy feels each Monday, Wednesday, and Friday goes. Our usual pattern is wait to be called to lab for blood work, wait to be called for vital signs to be taken, wait even longer for the test results to come back, and wait for test results review with either a PA or NP. We hold our breath at that point to see if we have to wait further for any fluids or platelets to be infused. Wash, rinse, repeat. But I do have to say that overall, Judy is doing extremely well with the Jakafi treatment. We should finish up the round of pills next Wednesday. She is scheduled for a bone marrow biopsy that day as well as review with Dr. Ravandi and the research team. Lots of decisions to make after the results of the bone marrow biopsy come back.

But I'd like to say something about the wait time that I've observed. In this waiting room full of strangers thrown together by damnable diseases, there are certain looks that caregivers give other caregivers. There are certain looks that cancer fighters give other cancer fighters. It's a forged bond among complete strangers that says…I know what you're dealing with, I know the fears you're facing, I know the struggles you're trying to balance, and a hundred other glances that are completely understood by people on the same path. So…how do I approach the wait times? Talk & laugh. Reach out with a smile and a nod. Use words if they seem appropriate. Get to know others from different areas of the world. Houston has always been a multi-cultural city and the waiting room is a great snapshot that reflects that.

So…we wait and we nod and we laugh and we tear up with other kindred folk walking similar but different paths. We try to spread the love of Christ, sometimes with words, sometimes without. And we pray that the message that we have eternal hope gets across. Coram DEO

So…my question is this…if you knew that you only had 30 days remaining on earth, how would you approach each day? Would you smile more? Would you spend more time with loved ones? Would you reach out to someone you don't know in hopes of getting to understand them better? Would you give more? Would you know without a doubt where you would spend eternity? What would you do?

Go do that today. Love y'all. Coram DEO

Chapter Sixteen – April 2018

04.14.2018 Update

It's been a year since Judy's Journey here on earth was completed and she stepped into eternity. Into the very presence of the One Whom she adored. The One she wanted so much for her friends and family to know as she did…as her personal Lord and Savior.

It's been a year of ups and downs for me as you can probably imagine; but certainly more ups than downs. It's been a year where I've found myself single again, widowed, or other (depending on the information card you fill out) after 37 years of marriage. The first time I marked 'Widowed' it really hit me. I've learned to cope with the grief by attending a Community Grief Support Group for a 10 week session and truly gained depth of insight that has allowed me to move forward. Not to move on as there will always be the wonderful memories and years that we had together. Years of growth together, years of raising our children together, three moves together, youth ministry together, building friendships together, struggling together, community service together.

It was a year of reflection as to what do I do now? I had the house remodeled with design input from my daughter-in-love, Charlie, and my daughter, Jennifer. The only requirement was the house could NOT look like an 80's fraternity house. Man…did they ever hit it completely out of the ballpark. Neighbors continue to stop by to say what a beautiful transformation it is. Judy and I had a long list of things that needed to be done as most homeowners do. Well…the list is complete and I think Judy would be well pleased. I've also started back to work two days a week and mentally things seem to be going well. On Wednesday nights I'm a member of the Hospitality Staff serving meals to our church members and I truly love it.

The biggest part of the reflection involves remembering the sweet prayers of our friends and church family that sustained me through the past year as well as texts, lunch invitations, telephone calls, emails, Facebook posts and visits. I have been and continue to be a truly blessed man.

Thank You to my Lord and Savior, Jesus Christ, for loving me through the past years. It is in Him that I place my faith and trust.

It is well with my soul.

Coram DEO

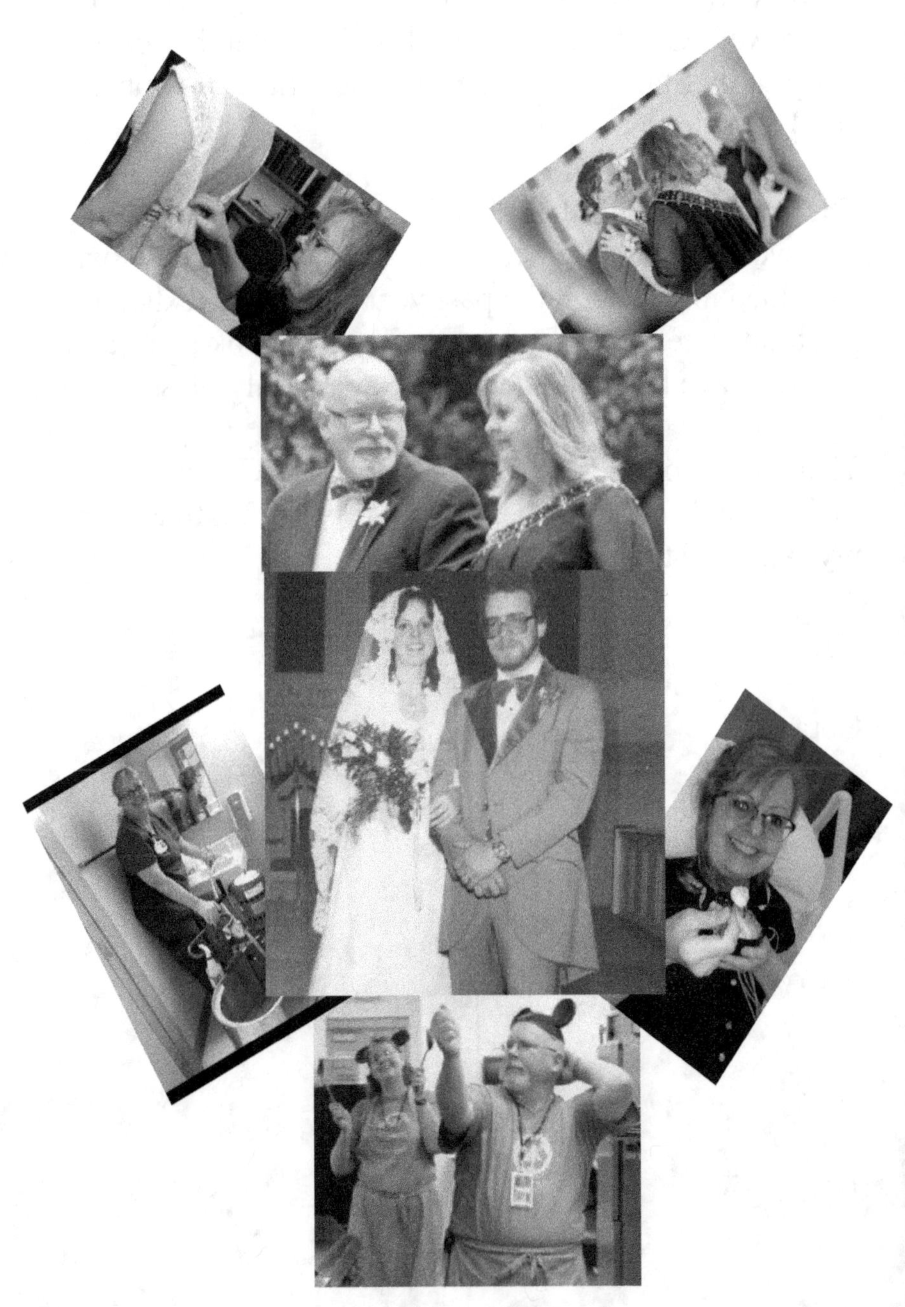

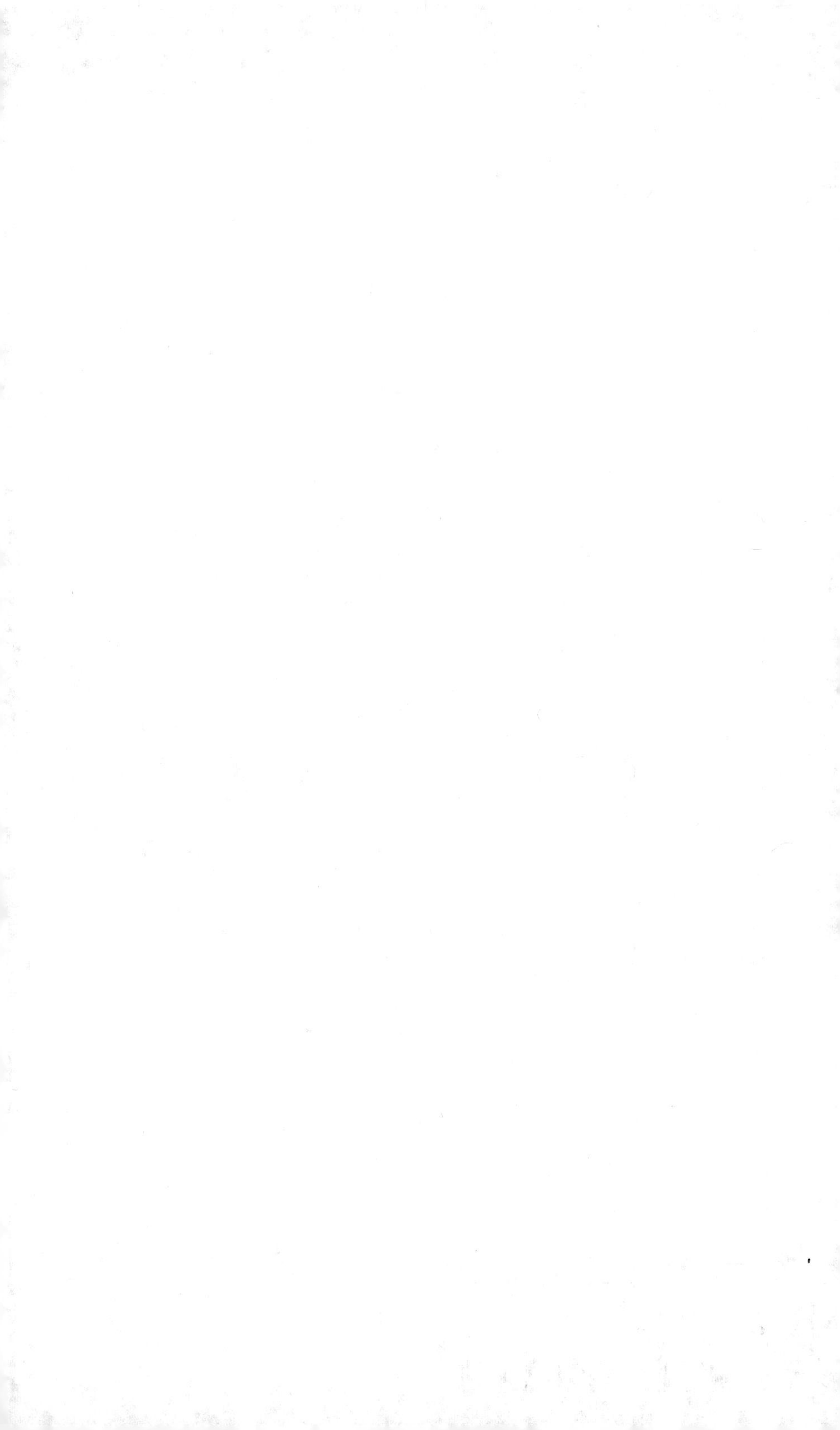